Musculoskeletal Injection Skills

This book is dedicated to Rod, Clive and Barbara

Musculoskeletal Injection Skills

Monica Kesson MScGrad DipPhys MCSP CertEd CertFE

Elaine Atkins DProf MA GradDipPhys MCSP CertFE

Ian Davies MB ChB

Foreword by
Richard Ellis

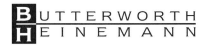

EDINBURGH LONDON NEW YORK PHILADELPHIA ST LOUIS SYDNEY TORONTO 2002

BUTTERWORTH-HEINEMANN
An imprint of Elsevier Science Limited

First published 2002

ISBN 07506 43722

British Library Cataloguing in Publication Data
A catalogue record for this book is available from the British Library

Library of Congress Cataloging in Publication Data
A catalog record for this book is available from the Library of Congress

Note
Medical knowledge is constantly changing. As new information becomes available, changes in treatment, procedures, equipment and the use of drugs become necessary. The authors and the publishers have taken care to ensure that the information given in this text is accurate and up to date. However, readers are strongly advised to confirm that the information, especially with regard to drug usage, complies with the latest legislation and standards of practice.

 your source for books, journals and multimedia in the health sciences
www.elsevierhealth.com

The publisher's policy is to use paper manufactured from sustainable forests

Printed in China by RDC Group Limited

Contents

About the authors

Monica Kesson and Elaine Atkins are both physiotherapists in private practice who share a commitment to the development of the educational course of the Society of Orthopaedic Medicine. As educators they both have a gift for making the complicated clear and this was reflected in their previous collaborative best selling publication 'Orthopaedic Medicine – a Practical Approach' (1998). Ian Davies is a general practitioner and teacher of orthopaedic medicine, who also achieved an anaesthetic fellowship earlier in his medical career. He was the prime mover in developing the Society's Injection Module to provide comprehensive training for physiotherapists keen to develop their skills in this relatively new specialism within physiotherapy. All three authors support a multi-disciplinary approach to primary care and extended scope of practice within physiotherapy. This has underpinned their determination to produce a text that is relevant to both medical practitioners and physiotherapists alike.

Foreword

Dr Richard Ellis

What's the difference between a bible and an encyclopaedia? To my mind a bible is a friendly companion that I constantly refer to, whereas an encyclopaedia is a mine of information that I never quite get round to looking up. So, a bible is something by my side, which keeps me on the straight and narrow, allowing me as far as possible to live a purposeful and rewarding life.

'Musculoskeletal Injection Skills' is certainly a bible. It contains not only the primary information about how to position your patient and yourself for all the common musculoskeletal injections, but also answers those doubts and little ignorances which nag most of us who want to do the best for our patients. If you're starting from scratch, this book will keep you as free as possible from these nags. And in addition, when you dip into it in an (unusual) idle moment, or it opens at a page you hadn't intended, there are yet more pearls of information revealed.

What a refreshing concept this book is, also. In the 'corporate structure' which medicine often seems to have, each division, such as 'pharmacology' and 'musculoskeletal medicine' is liable to remain quite separate with its own textbook and jargon; as exactly may the disciplines, such as 'doctoring' and 'physiotherapy'. Here we are dealing with a clinical task, with its basic evidence of efficacy, which the book takes apart into its essential aspects from basic sciences through to the clinical scenario and complications. The patient who is needing an injection wants it to be done by someone who has all the knowledge in this book: and the label on the operator's collar is not important.

Of course extra background knowledge, as the book states, is of the greatest assistance on the diagnostic side, and familiarity with the applied anatomy and the function and dysfunction of the neuromusculoskeletal system is essential. You must have an understanding both of these areas and with the contents of this book if you are able to be an efficient and safe injector in orthopaedic medicine, whether you are physiotherapist or doctor.

Acknowledgements

Dr James Cyriax will always deserve acknowledgement for his life's work that provided the approach that underpins this text.

We are grateful to Butterworth Heinemann for providing the impetus to produce 'Musculoskeletal Injection Skills'. Heidi Allen and Caroline Makepeace have been supportive throughout and we have appreciated their understanding when schedules have gone awry.

The photographs and illustrations have been supported by an educational grant from Pfizer Ltd and Pharmacia Ltd.

The Council of the Society of Orthopaedic Medicine has continued to stand behind us and thanks are due particularly to those Society Fellows who suggested changes: Dr Gordon Cameron, Paul Hattam, Alison Smeatham, Gordon Smith and Dr Bruce Thompson.

Our colleagues within our respective practices have been unstinting with their support, gamely keeping things going through times of literary turbulence. We are also indebted to our friends for providing a much needed social oasis.

As ever, those at home deserve the most special of thanks for providing inspiration, admiration and encouragement. Thank you Rod, Andrew, Denise; Clive, Kate, Tess; and Barbara.

Preface

Musculoskeletal medicine and therapy have traditionally sat side be side, with both medical practitioners and physiotherapists combining experience in the assessment and clinical diagnosis of musculoskeletal lesions and applying their different approaches and skills.

The role of Dr James Cyriax was pivotal in the development of orthopaedic medicine, arguably the bedrock of musculoskeletal medicine. The specialism developed from his background in orthopaedic surgery at St Thomas' Hospital, London, in 1929, where he was intrigued by conditions presenting in orthopaedic clinics with normal radiographic findings, where the lesion was clearly within the so-called 'soft tissues'. Putting surgery aside, he devoted his life's work to developing a system for examining the soft tissues towards establishing a clinical diagnosis, and from there to devising treatment techniques for the lesions diagnosed. Throughout his long professional life, he dedicated himself to the continued development of the specialism and, as well as techniques of mobilisation, manipulation and traction, injections were very much part of his treatment approach to the soft tissue lesions encountered within clinical practice. His approach was bi-disciplinary from the outset, drawing on the experience of medical practitioners and physiotherapists and acknowledging the importance of co-operation and collaboration in the management of patients. Medical practitioners and physiotherapists were taught alongside each other on his educational courses to acquire the theory and skills of assessment, manual techniques and injection therapy, even though the boundaries of scope of practice prevented physiotherapists from being able to put injection skills into practice. Musculoskeletal injections, therefore, traditionally remained firmly within the province of the physician.

Physiotherapy is derived from a base of massage, remedial gymnastics and electrotherapy (Williams, 1986) and these have traditionally been considered to be the core skills of the profession, in determining scope of practice.

The Chartered Society of Physiotherapy (CSP), the professional body of physiotherapy, is responsible for both the training and support of Chartered Physiotherapists whilst having a key role in deciding professional issues. A discussion document published in 'Physiotherapy' in 1988 ('Physiotherapy', August 1988, pp 356–358) emphasised the process of developing practice. It was clear in its guidelines for exploring developments in practice that the 'new modality, technique or philosophy' should be 'clearly based upon the core of physiotherapy'. This dictum had presented the stumbling block for the introduction of the use of injections which had been first considered in 1987 ('Physiotherapy', April 1990, pp 218–219), when the Professional Practice Committee of the CSP recommended that the giving of injections by physiotherapists, as an invasive technique, was not within the scope of physiotherapy practice.

It was also highlighted that the administration of drugs by physiotherapists was not consistent with Section 58(2)(b) of the Medicines Act 1968, where only registered medical practitioners, dentists and veterinary surgeons have the right to prescribe drugs, and that 'such a practice could cause conflict between physiotherapists and doctors' ('Physiotherapy', April 1990, pp 218–219).

With the continued development of autonomy within physiotherapy came the extended role of the profession in orthopaedics and rheumatology, where orthopaedic and rheumatology 'assistants' or 'practitioners' were being created, whose role included the administration of local steroid injection, with consultant support but without direct intervention. This move towards greater autonomy was welcomed by both the medical and physiotherapy professions as a safe and cost-effective use of resources (Hourigan and Weatherley, 1994).

Hockin and Bannister (1994) examined the extended role of a physiotherapist in an outpatient orthopaedic clinic and in analysing the treatments selected in patient management identified that 22% of patients had received local steroid injection. With the existence of such a fait accompli and the moves of continuing professional development in encouraging the process of developing practice towards skill specialism (Bergman, 1990), the CSP Professional Practice Committee was pressed to extend the scope of practice of physiotherapy to include injections in December 1995. The CSP produced guidelines for practice, which clearly enforced the need for proper post-graduate training. With respect to the Medicines Act it was pronounced that the medical practitioner would be responsible for prescribing the drug but the physiotherapist would be responsible for administering the injection.

In interpreting the term 'proper post-graduate training' a vehicle was required that would extend the physiotherapists' existing knowledge in injection therapy and allow the development of skills in the use of this modality. Even for physiotherapists who had been taught, and were experienced in, the application of the principles and practice of orthopaedic medicine and musculoskeletal therapy, it was apparent that further training was required to be able to achieve both the competence and confidence to inject.

'Bolt on' courses in injection therapy have been developed that rely on a sound existing knowledge of functional anatomy and clinical diagnosis of soft tissue lesions, with an awareness of the basic tenets of injection therapy. There are particular implications for the process of clinical reasoning, now that injections have come to form part of the armoury of the manual therapist and care in the selection of this invasive technique and issues of clinical safety have been emphasised within the training programmes.

Evidence based medicine has been a driver in consolidating the basis for selection of treatments applied in medicine and physiotherapy. In 1999, the CSP endorsed 'A Clinical Guideline for the Use of Injection Therapy by Physiotherapists' that was prepared by the Association of Chartered Physiotherapists in Orthopaedic Medicine (ACPOM), a clinical interest group of the CSP. The guideline was rigorous in its approach to identifying evidence to support its recommendations for best practice in the application of injection therapy, and as well as being pertinent to physiotherapists intending to use the modality, it is also relevant to medical practitioners who work in the field of musculoskeletal medicine and for general practitioners in primary care. At the time of writing, the guideline is undergoing a process of clinical audit to be able to monitor the extent to which it is being followed and to enhance reflection on the effectiveness of injection therapy in clinical practice.

The Crown Review of Prescribing, Supply and Administration of Medicines (1999) recommended that prescribing rights should be extended to physiotherapists, with appropriate legislation affecting physiotherapists, pharmacists and other health professionals awaiting Parliamentary discussion time ('Frontline', April 2000, p 7). Dr June Crown, who headed the review, cited extended scope practitioners as one professional group that should be eligible for independent prescriber status. This would allow appropriately qualified physiotherapists to prescribe and administer drugs having made a diagnosis and devised a treatment plan. The extended role of physiotherapy practitioners working in musculoskeletal clinics has already been demonstrated to be effective in the primary care setting, (Hattam and Smeatham, 1999) and the role will undoubtedly be enhanced still further by the introduction of prescribing rights, albeit limited at the outset.

Injection therapy courses sit comfortably within master's programmes since they conform to the achievement of Level 4 (master's level) learning outcomes in allowing the demonstration of mastery in the application of a clinical skill within post-graduate education programmes. Clinical reasoning is paramount in the selection of intra-articular and intralesional injections as appropriate and efficacious treatment techniques. Subsequent evaluation and reflection on treatment outcomes promotes safe and effective practice.

This text aims to support courses in injection therapy by addressing the theory underpinning the approach and the specific techniques presented on a regional basis. It will also be pertinent to those medical practitioners who find themselves new to the specialism of musculoskeletal medicine, or will act as a refresher or corroborative reference to those who have existing experience. Physiotherapy 'grandfathers' who have been using the modality for many years, and who have now been able to own up to the skill, may also be included within the latter group.

The adopted title 'Musculoskeletal Injection Skills' is intended to encompass those injections that may be appropriate for peripheral lesions encountered in sports and orthopaedic medicine, and is in line with the increasingly popular use of the terms musculoskeletal medicine and therapy within the respective professions. We have included the injection techniques that are credited to the original work of Cyriax but have been developed and added to in the global domain of orthopaedic medicine. We have aimed for clarity and accuracy in presentation, continuing with the style of superimposing key points of anatomy onto the original photographs, as used in a previous collaborative publication provided by Pfizer Pharmaceuticals, 'Joint Injection Techniques, a User's Guide', (1996), but with impressive enhancement through the artistry and technical brilliance of our medical illustrator.

All who use injections within their clinical practice acknowledge the need for continued research to monitor this developing therapy, and especially to evaluate its efficacy with respect to other available treatment modalities in both medicine and physiotherapy. We support this research wholeheartedly, and would guide the reader to the research grants available from the Society of Orthopaedic Medicine, and its collaborative post-graduate programmes, to support prospective researchers in their endeavours (see below). 'Musculoskeletal Injection Skills' aims to be an important foundation for both clinical practice and future investigation in injection therapy.

Monica Kesson, Elaine Atkins and Ian Davies

Society of Orthopaedic Medicine

(Registered charity: 802164)

Administrative Director:

Amanda Sherwood
PO Box 223
Patchway
Bristol
BS32 4XD

AmandaSherwood@compuserve.com

www.soc-ortho-med.org

1 Principles of musculoskeletal injections

Introduction to Section 1

This section presents the theory underpinning the administration of intra-articular and intralesional injections for peripheral musculoskeletal lesions. The first two chapters provide an overview of basic pharmacology and the essential equipment required for administering injections. Safety precautions are highlighted with guidance on recognizing and dealing with emergency situations. The third chapter describes injectable drugs for use in musculoskeletal injections, with important notes on their mechanism of action, effects and side effects. The section concludes with a chapter on general principles of injection therapy and lists the indications and contraindications for injections, while explaining the application of general techniques, and providing notes on record-keeping. A flow chart provides a background for the clinical decision-making process.

1 Basic pharmacology – what do drugs do?

CHAPTER SUMMARY

This chapter presents the key points of pharmacology that are relevant to applied injection therapy. Pharmacology is introduced with an outline of how drugs are administered, absorbed, distributed, metabolized and eliminated. Drug nomenclature is then defined.

The pharmacology presented in this chapter is basic, for which we make no apology. In preparing a text to enable both medical practitioners and physiotherapists to enhance their injection skills, the authors were mindful of the lack of pharmacology within undergraduate physiotherapy training, at least until relatively recently when injections came within the scope of physiotherapy practice in 1995.

All will agree that an understanding of pharmacology or, simplistically, how drugs work, is essential for the application of injection therapy. Medical practitioners may choose to skip to Chapter 2, where the theory presented in Chapter 1 will be assumed, and all should be equal from there on.

A **drug** is a substance which modifies body function (Grundy 1990, Kalant 1998). **Pharmacology** is the study of drugs and their action in the body. It can be subdivided into **pharmacokinetics** – the process whereby drugs are absorbed, distributed, metabolized and eliminated from the body or, simply, what the body does with the drug – and **pharmacodynamics** – the action of drugs on the cells, tissues and organs or, simply, what the drug does to the body (Grundy 1990, Rang et al 1995, Laurence et al 1997). For a drug to be therapeutically useful it must act selectively on particular cells and tissues, i.e. the target for the drug action. Individual classes of drugs bind to certain targets and individual targets recognize certain classes of drugs. However, a drug is not usually completely specific in its action and its effects on cells and tissues other than the target inevitably produce side effects (Rang et al 1995).

THE PHARMACOKINETIC PROCESS

In order to produce its effects, a drug must be present in appropriate concentrations at the target tissue (Benet 1996). As mentioned above, the pharmacokinetic process (what the body does with the drug) is the process whereby a drug is absorbed, distributed, metabolized and eliminated from the body. In order to go through these processes the drug must first cross the cell membrane. The cell membrane preserves and regulates the internal environment and consists of bilayers of lipid molecules with 'islands' of proteins (Laurence et al 1997).

A variety of different mechanisms enable the drug to cross cell membranes within the tissues to facilitate its absorption. The drug's molecular size, its relative solubility in lipid and water, its ionization and other properties, can all influence absorption (Kalant 1998). There is a close correlation between the permeability of the cell membrane and the drug's solubility in lipid and water, and for this reason lipid solubility is an important determinant of the pharmacokinetic characteristics of a drug. The relative solubility determines whether the drug molecule will stay in the water phase or permeate the fatty cell membrane. Generally, a more lipid-soluble drug molecule is less water-soluble and a less lipid-soluble drug molecule is more water-soluble. Properties such as the rate of absorption, penetration into the tissues and duration of action can be predicted from knowledge of the drug's lipid-solubility (Rang et al 1995).

Drug absorption

In whatever form a drug is given, it will first pass into free solution at the site of administration. If administered by mouth, the dissolved drug is absorbed into the portal circulation (the visceral system which circulates via the liver). If administered by injection, inhalation or via the skin or mucous membranes, it is directly absorbed into the systemic circulation. Musculoskeletal injections are intended to directly affect the target tissue, but some systemic absorption is inevitable and is responsible for unwanted side effects (*see* Chapter 3).

Absorption is the passage of the drug from its administration site into the plasma, which then transports it to its site of action or elimination (Rang et al 1995). The more rapidly the drug is absorbed the more rapidly it is eliminated, and factors which affect its absorption therefore also affect its duration of action. Relatively insoluble drugs, e.g. triamcinolone acetonide, have a longer period of action than relatively soluble drugs such as hydrocortisone.

The drug may pass through some tissues and organs which are not affected by it, but act as reservoirs affecting the drug's overall volume distribution and concentration in the plasma. Some drugs act as agonists (activators) binding to specific receptors on or in the target cells. A small number of drugs act as antagonists (causing no activation or acting as blockers), binding to a receptor without initiating change, but preventing other substances from gaining access to the receptor.

Drug administration routes

The main administration routes are:

- oral
- sublingual
- buccal
- rectal
- topical – by application to the epithelial surfaces, e.g. skin, cornea
- inhalation
- injection

For the purposes of this text, administration by injection is the only route that concerns us. Injections are delivered:

- intravenously
- subcutaneously
- intramuscularly
- intralesionally
- intra-articularly

Intravenous injections

Intravenous injection gives direct access to the circulation and is the fastest route of delivery, producing high concentrations of the drug. It is initially delivered principally to organs of high blood-flow such as the brain, liver, heart, lungs, and kidneys. It is an appropriate route for the administration of lidocaine to treat cardiac arrhythmias, but not for musculoskeletal injections where the high blood levels produced can be dangerous. Musculoskeletal injections require local, not systemic, effects. The rate at which the injection is given determines the levels of drug in the circulation, with a rapid intravenous injection producing the highest blood levels. The disadvantage of the intravenous route is that if the drug is delivered too quickly, the plasma concentration rises so rapidly that the normal mechanisms of distribution are outpaced and toxic side-effects can occur (Laurence et al 1997, BNF 2000).

Subcutaneous, intramuscular, intralesional or intra-articular injections

These types of injections produce a slower effect than the intravenous route, but generally a quicker effect than the oral route. The subcutaneous route tends to have relatively poor absorption and repeated injections into one site can cause fat atrophy (lipotrophy) (Laurence et al 1997). Absorption may be more rapid by the intramuscular route, which is suitable particularly for irritant drugs and depot preparations (slow-release drugs that may remain in the tissues for days, weeks or months).

CLINICAL TIP: Anatomical knowledge of the structures to be injected is paramount. A poorly placed injection into the subcutaneous tissues may cause fat atrophy (lipotrophy), as may be seen with injection at the tennis elbow site.

Musculoskeletal injections are delivered to the exact site of the lesion, in order to produce their effects locally, but some of the drug may be absorbed into the general circulation. As mentioned above, complete specificity cannot be guaranteed, and knowledge of the side effects of the injected drugs is therefore most important. The recognized side effects will be covered under the topics of local anaesthetics and corticosteroids (*see* Chapter 3).

CLINICAL TIP: Take care, a rapid, accidental intravenous injection of local anaesthetic can produce life-threatening side effects. Therefore, when delivering an intralesional injection containing local anaesthetic, aspirate before delivery of the solution to ensure that placement of the needle is not within a blood vessel.

The rate of absorption of the drug from the intralesional site will depend on:

- the nature of the tissue injected
- local blood-flow
- the rate of diffusion through the tissues
- the solubility of the preparation

A high local blood-flow produces more rapid absorption, but this will vary according to the tissue injected, as some tissues are more vascular than others. The rate of diffusion is generally more rapid in inflamed tissues due to the increased blood-flow in the area. The more soluble the preparation injected, the more rapidly it is absorbed.

Drug distribution

Distribution of the drug to its target occurs by passage across cell membranes and via the body fluids by:

- diffusion
- filtration
- carrier molecules

Diffusion

Diffusion is the natural tendency of any substance to move from an area of high concentration to one of low concentration. Corticosteroids are transported across cell membranes by this method. Lipid-soluble substances diffuse more readily into cells and this is the most important way in which a drug enters the tissues to be distributed through them. Drugs show greater or lesser degrees of lipid-solubility according to the structural properties of the molecule and the acidity or alkalinity of the environment (Laurence et al 1997). Local anaesthetics are weak bases (i.e. alkaline) and are less soluble in lipids in an acid environment, such as within inflamed tissues. They therefore do not cross cell membranes easily and their activity becomes impaired. However, in an alkaline environment, local anaesthetics are comparatively more soluble in lipids, and cross the cell membrane more readily by diffusion.

Filtration

Filtration is the passage of small water-soluble molecules through aqueous channels in tight junctions between adjacent epithelial cells. Filtration plays a minor role in drug distribution and is mainly concerned with excretion of drugs by glomerular filtration (Laurence et al 1997).

Carrier molecules

Carrier molecules are special protein molecules within the lipid bilayer, which act as 'ferry boats' allowing drug molecules, which are insufficiently lipid-soluble to penetrate lipid membranes on their own, to cross by active transportation against or with the concentration gradient (Rang et al 1995, Laurence et al 1997).

Drug metabolism

Drugs affect the metabolic processes of the cell in a variety of ways, such as by blocking ion channels, e.g. the blocking action of local anaesthetics on the voltage-gated sodium channel, or by inhibiting the action of enzymes. Specific receptors (proteins) may exist within the cell to which a drug may become bound (Rang et al 1995).

Most drugs are treated by the body as foreign substances (xenobiotics) and are metabolized by enzymes (Rang et al 1995, Laurence et al 1997). This process occurs mainly in the liver, but other tissues such as the kidneys, gut mucosa, or lungs may contribute.

Metabolism occurs in two phases, involving different types of biochemical reaction (Rang et al 1995, Laurence et al 1997):

- An initial 'phase I reaction', which changes the drug molecule by oxidation, reduction or hydrolysis, producing a derivative which may be more active or toxic than the original drug. In some cases the original drug (known as a pro-drug) is inactive and the phase I metabolite is in fact the active drug.
- The subsequent 'phase II reaction', which usually terminates the drug's activity producing an inactive compound.

Excretion of drugs

Once a drug is absorbed it must be eliminated from the body and this normally begins with a process of metabolic intervention. Most drugs are excreted as metabolites but a few are eliminated unchanged.

One method of describing the rate of elimination is by the concept of the **'plasma half life'** $(t_{1/2})$ of the drug, which is the time taken for the plasma concentration to fall by 50%. In reality this is an oversimplification, e.g. with a slowly absorbed drug such as the corticosteroid triamcinolone acetonide, absorption is still taking place as elimination occurs. The uneven distribution of some drugs throughout the fluid compartments and tissues of the body makes the concept an inaccurate measure. The plasma half-life is only one factor involved in the duration of action of a drug, e.g. dexamethasone has a longer half-life compared with triamcinolone, but the available preparation of dexamethasone is shorter acting, due to its greater solubility than the available preparations of triamcinolone.

As mentioned above, there are three main routes of elimination:

- The main route is via the kidneys, where the drug and its metabolites leave the plasma by filtration through minute pores in the capillary walls of the glomerulus.
- The lungs deal with inhalational agents such as general anaesthetics.
- Some drugs and their metabolites are excreted in the bile by the liver, and ultimately eliminated in the faeces. Reabsorption is common in the gut, making this a relatively inefficient route of elimination, but 25% of corticosteroids are excreted in this way.

THE PHARMACODYNAMIC PROCESS

Pharmacodynamics is the action of drugs on the cells, tissues and organs of the body, or what the drug does to the body. Drugs act by altering the body's control systems. Most bind to a specialized constituent of the cell to alter its function, selectively changing the physiological or pathological system to which it contributes. Drugs may act on the cell membrane, or may affect the metabolic processes within and outside the cell (Laurence et al 1997). Further information on the pharmacodynamic processes of injectable drugs used in musculoskeletal medicine will be covered in Chapter 3.

DRUG NOMENCLATURE

Each drug has three names:

- The **chemical name** is of no clinical interest but describes the compound for the chemist, e.g. N-diethylaminoacetyl-2, 6 xylidine hydrochloride monohydrate, which is the chemical name for lidocaine hydrochloride (Wood-Smith et al 1968).
- The **generic name** or approved name is chosen by the Nomenclature Committee of the British Pharmacopoeia Commission (Henry 1991), e.g. lidocaine (now the internationally standardized name for lignocaine), or triamcinolone acetonide.
- The **proprietary or trade name** is chosen by the manufacturer and may apply only to a specific formulation, e.g. Xylocaine® (lidocaine manufactured by Astra Pharmaceuticals), Adcortyl® (triamcinolone acetonide suspension 10 mg/ml manufactured by ER Squibb & Sons), Kenalog® (triamcinolone acetonide suspension 40 mg/ml manufactured by ER Squibb & Sons).

Since proprietary names differ internationally, generic prescribing is the preferred method for clarity, economy and convenience (Laurence et al 1997).

CONCLUSION

This chapter has been deliberate in its attempt to set out the basic pharmacology of how drugs work. From that starting point, the next step will be to consider the equipment needed and the safety precautions to be taken prior to performing an injection. These topics will form the basis of the following chapter.

2 Essential equipment, safety precautions and emergency situations

CHAPTER SUMMARY

This chapter provides details of the range of needle and syringe sizes commonly used for musculoskeletal injections. Emphasis is placed on precautions to be taken to ensure safety and to minimize the risk of infection. The potential side effects are listed, with notes on how to recognize and deal with emergency situations.

BASIC EQUIPMENT

Drug containers

Drugs for injection are usually supplied in either vials or ampoules (Fig. 2.1). Vials have a rubber cap, which is designed to be penetrated by the needle and to self-seal afterwards. The cap may be covered by a hard plastic seal (e.g. Kenalog®, Depomedrone®) or by a metal seal. Ampoules are normally of glass construction, with no separate stopper, and care needs to be taken to prevent injury when breaking off the top. The narrow neck of the ampoule may be scored during manufacture or a file may be used to weaken the neck to facilitate opening. Lidocaine and some other local anaesthetics may be contained in plastic ampoules such as Polyamps™ or Sure-amps™. Each usually comes with full instructions but generally the top of the ampoule twists off and the syringe taper then fits directly into the neck of the ampoule.

▶ **FIGURE 2.1**

Containers of drugs in common use for musculoskeletal injections (as mentioned in the previous chapter, lidocaine is now the internationally standardized name for lignocaine – at the time of writing the drug was still being issued in containers using the traditional labelling of 'lignocaine', as pictured).

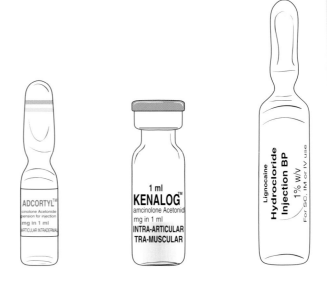

CLINICAL TIP: Caution should be exercised to prevent inflicting skin wounds if a glass ampoule should shatter on opening. An opening device should be used or the hands protected with a cloth or gloves.

Syringes

Disposable syringes should be used (Fig. 2.2). These are all manufactured with expiry dates clearly marked on the paper side of the wrapper. This wrapping is usually of 'peel apart' type, consisting of paper and clear plastic.

Sizes of 1, 2, 5, 10, 20, 30, 50 and 60 ml are available, and generally speaking the size is chosen to be appropriate for the amount of solution delivered. More pressure may be required when injecting the teno-osseous sites of tendons, e.g. the common extensor tendon at the elbow (tennis elbow/enthesitis). This can be achieved by using a small piston to produce a higher pressure for a given force and a 1 ml syringe is ideal for this. The effect of syringe size on injection pressure is illustrated below (Fig. 2.3).

Needles

Disposable needles should be used (Fig. 2.4). These are packed in 'peel apart' paper and clear plastic with the needle protected by a rigid or semi-rigid plastic tube. All should be clearly marked with the size of the needle and sterilization and expiry dates on the paper side of the wrapper. The needles are available in a range of lengths and diameters but it is common practice to refer to the colour of the plastic hub, which denotes the diameter (or gauge) of the needle.

▶ **FIGURE 2.2**

Syringes in common use for musculoskeletal injections.

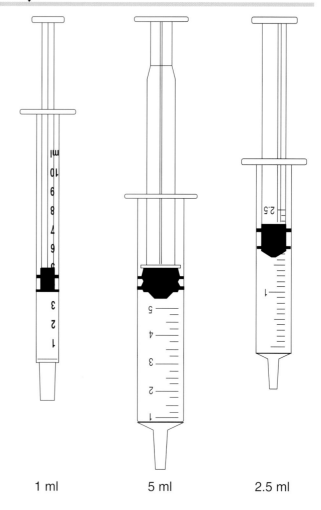

1 ml   5 ml   2.5 ml

▶ **FIGURE 2.3**

Effect of the syringe size on injection pressure.

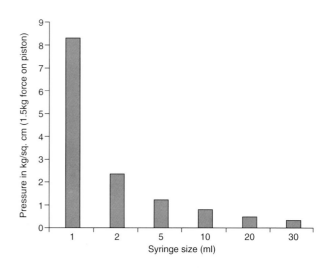

Needles in common use for
musculoskeletal injections.

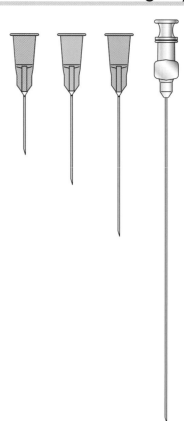

Table 2.1 gives an indication of the needle sizes available; those highlighted in bold type denote the needles more commonly used in musculoskeletal injections.

For some musculoskeletal injections a spinal needle may be an appropriate choice (e.g. hip joint or psoas bursa injections) and although available in varying lengths, these are generally longer than the standard hypodermic needles (e.g. 20G × 3½″, 0.9 × 90 mm). Spinal needles have a wire stylet which remains present in the lumen of the needle during its insertion, to prevent the skin being taken in with the needle, and is withdrawn before connecting the syringe. This feature is important for spinal injections but is also pertinent when the needle is required for musculoskeletal injections, since that fragment of skin may be a means of carrying infection to the site of the lesion.

Table 2.1   Needle sizes and hub colours (G = gauge)

	Imperial size (inches)	Metric size (mm)	Hub colour
Fine diameter	**25G × 5/8″**	**0.5 × 16 mm**	**Orange**
	25G × 1″	0.5 × 25 mm	Orange
	23G × 1″	**0.6 × 25 mm**	**Blue**
	23G × 1¼″	0.6 × 30 mm	Blue
	21G × 1½″	**0.8 × 40 mm**	**Green**
	21G × 2″	0.8 × 50 mm	Green
Large diameter	19G × 1½″	1.1 × 40 mm	White

The needles and syringes referred to above are usually available from NHS supplies for general practitioners, or may be ordered from a pharmacy or medical supplier for physiotherapists or medical practitioners in private practice.

DISPOSAL OF EQUIPMENT

'Sharps' containers should be used for the disposal of syringes, needles and empty drug containers. These containers will be readily available in hospitals or general practitioners' surgeries, where a policy will be in place for the safe disposal of 'sharps'. In private clinics, advice should be sought from the local council's environmental health department, who can usually provide suitable containers and offer a disposal service.

GENERAL SAFETY PRECAUTIONS

All medical practitioners and physiotherapists wishing to practise injection therapy should undergo a course of immunization against hepatitis B. This involves three doses, the second being given 1 month after the first and the third given 6 months after the first. An accelerated regime is possible should it be required (contact your general practitioner or practice nurse for further details).

Antibody levels should be checked 2–4 months after completing the course, with 80–90% of people responding overall. Those over 40 years-of-age are less likely to respond. As a general rule, poor responders should receive a booster dose and non-responders should consider repeating the course. All responders should probably have a booster dose after 5 years (Salisbury & Begg 1996).

You should be aware of all safety policies within your place of work relating to protection against viruses (hepatitis B, HIV). Medical practitioners and physiotherapists working in private clinics may need to establish a policy for themselves.

All equipment should be disposed of safely (see above). Clinical waste should be placed in appropriately marked plastic bags (usually yellow) and removed for subsequent incineration (seek advice from appropriate local environmental health department). Spilt blood or body fluids should be dealt with correctly using latex gloves and paper towels. If gloves are to be worn, latex is safer than polythene for protection against viruses (Korniewicz et al 1989). The area of spillage should be cleaned with sodium hypochlorite solution, e.g. Domestos™, rinsing any soiled linen in cold water and an appropriate disinfectant, e.g. 1 in 10 solution of bleach.

Needlestick injuries

To prevent needlestick injuries, a used needle should never be re-sheathed. However, if an injury does occur, the recommended procedure is to encourage bleeding as much as possible and to wash with soap and water. Urgent medical advice may be obtained by telephone from the following sources as appropriate **(Salisbury & Begg 1996):**

- the nearest Public Health Laboratory
- the Consultant in Public Health Medicine (CPHM) on call for the Local Health Board in Scotland
- a hospital Control of Infection Officer
- the occupational health services

CLINICAL TIP: Remember – **NEVER** re-sheath a used needle!

'No-touch' technique

A 'no-touch', 'clean' technique is vitally important, particularly when using corticosteroid agents, since their immunosuppressive effect increases susceptibility to infection and makes infection more difficult to detect and treat (Schimmer & George 1998). When injecting a joint, septic arthritis should be considered as a serious, but avoidable, complication.

Possible sources of infection include:

- skin organisms carried in during the injection procedure or spread from other adjacent infections
- introduction via contaminated equipment or solutions
- haematogenous spread from distant infection such as septicaemia, e.g. following dental procedures, or the use of genitourinary tract instrumentation as during cystoscopy
- direct trauma may have produced infection into the local area, particularly in superficial bursae, e.g. the prepatellar or olecranon bursae (Hughes 1996)

A 'no-touch' routine to minimize the risk of infection is suggested in Chapter 4.

Dosage safety margins

The recommended maximum dose for the local anaesthetic, lidocaine, is 200 mg (*see* Chapter 3). It is advised that to avoid reaching toxic levels of local anaesthetic, those new to musculoskeletal injection therapy may prefer to use no more than 5 ml of 1% lidocaine, or 15 ml of 0.5% lidocaine on one occasion. Local anaesthetics are relatively more toxic in more concentrated solutions and both figures given are deliberately below the maximum dose. These recommendations provide a wide safety margin to minimize the potential risk from accidental injection via a blood vessel directly into the bloodstream.

In general, the patient receives one injection for each musculoskeletal lesion diagnosed. In 1 year it is advisable not to give more than two injections into any one anatomical structure except the glenohumeral joint, where three may be necessary for the treatment of traumatic arthritis (frozen shoulder) (Kesson & Atkins 1998).

Should the patient present with more than one lesion, two injections could be considered at one treatment session, but it is recommended that the total dose of corticosteroid does not exceed 60 mg as a maximum, to err on the side of caution. However, if there is any query for particular drugs, the manufacturer's recommendation on the data sheet should be checked.

COMPLICATIONS AND DEALING WITH EMERGENCIES

Infection

It is not uncommon for patients undergoing corticosteroid injection to experience a post-injection flare of pain, which is treated by rest, ice and non-steroidal anti-inflammatory drugs, or simple analgesia. However, this must be distinguished from the pain signifying infection, which is generally more severe and lasts beyond the approximate limit of 72 hours of a post-injection flare. As mentioned above, corticosteroids can mask signs of infection, which are heat, redness, swelling and loss of function. If a septic arthritis or infection following intralesional injection is suspected, the patient should be referred urgently to hospital, where an initial aspiration to confirm diagnosis will be followed by intravenous antibiotic therapy (Hughes 1996).

Simple faint

This presents as pallor, hypotension with bradycardia, occasional twitching movements and possible eye-rolling. The normal management for such an event is to loosen tight clothing and to place the patient in a horizontal or lateral position with the feet raised. Most patients wake up as soon as they are horizontal, but if not they should be moved into the recovery position to safeguard the airway and to prevent the risk of aspiration should vomiting occur.

Allergy

This can vary from simple urticaria to anaphylaxis (see below). Urticaria may be present as a minor irritation or 'nettle rash' in which the itching may be treated with an antihistamine, e.g. Piriton®. A more severe urticaria may present as large wheals and possible facial and glossal swelling. Medical advice should be obtained for both situations but is urgent if facial or glossal swelling occurs. A rash other than that described above may present as an allergic dermatitis, for which the application of hydrocortisone cream may prove curative.

Anaphylactic shock

Anaphylaxis is described as a rapid, and often unanticipated, life-threatening syndrome triggered by a wide range of foreign substances and involving multiple organ systems (Brown 1995, Wyatt 1996). It is an extremely rare complication of injection, but requires prompt action to treat the laryngeal oedema, bronchospasm, hypotension and associated tachycardia (Apter & LaVallee 1994, BNF 2000).

An itchy sensation progressing rapidly to facial or glossal swelling, as mentioned for severe allergy above, may be an indication of impending anaphylactic shock. Should this event occur it should be treated as a medical emergency, physiotherapists should obtain urgent medical advice, and the routine for Basic Life Support should be followed (Gabbott & Baskett 1997, Handley 1997).

Following most regional anaesthetic procedures, maximum arterial plasma concentrations of anaesthetic develop within 10–25 minutes. For this reason, careful monitoring for toxic effects is recommended during the first 30 minutes after injection (CSP 1999, BNF 2000).

The CSP *Clinical Guideline for the Use of Injection Therapy by Physiotherapists* (CSP 1999) provides specific points for the management of anaphylactic shock, suggesting the following regime:

- stop delivery of the drug
- summon medical help
- administer adrenaline
- administer cardiopulmonary resuscitation

CONCLUSION

This chapter has provided details of the range of needle and syringe sizes commonly used for musculoskeletal injections. The precautions to be taken to ensure safety and to minimize the risk of infection have been highlighted. The potential side effects have been listed with important notes on how to recognize and deal with emergency situations. Chapter 3 will describe the drugs used in musculoskeletal injections, with information on their mechanism of action, effects and side effects.

3 Injectable drugs for musculoskeletal lesions

CHAPTER SUMMARY

This chapter sets out to provide an overview of the principal drugs used in musculoskeletal injections, with note of their mechanism of action, effects, side effects and contraindications. It contributes still further to the development of safe and effective practice in the administration of musculoskeletal injections.

CORTICOSTEROIDS

Local corticosteroid injections are used to reduce inflammation and pain, allowing mobilization. They are given intra-articularly to treat episodic disease flares, as in acute episodes of degenerative osteoarthrosis (e.g. osteoarthrosis of the knee), inflammatory arthritis (e.g. rheumatoid arthritis of the wrist) and occasionally traumatic arthritis (e.g. traumatic arthritis of the elbow) (Hunter & Blyth 1999).

Weitoft & Uddenfeldt (2000) suggested that the aspiration of synovial fluid before placement of an intra-articular injection of corticosteroid reduced the risk of relapse in patients with rheumatoid arthritis. Creamer (1999) reviewed the literature on the use of intra-articular corticosteroid injection in osteo-arthritis and noted several studies which indicated significant benefit compared with placebo in the knee, although the beneficial effects were short-lived.

Intralesional corticosteroid injections are given for tendinitis (e.g. tennis elbow), tenosynovitis (e.g. de Quervain's tenosynovitis), where the injection is delivered between the tendon and its sheath, compression neuropathies (e.g. carpal tunnel) and for some ligamentous lesions (e.g. coronary ligaments at the knee).

Corticosteroids are hormones that are produced in the body by the adrenal cortex. They are classified into two broad groups, mineralocorticoids and glucocorticoids. Although several individual corticosteroids have mixed actions, the main properties of the groups are:

- **mineralocorticoids** (the main endogenous hormone is aldosterone) influence water and electrolyte balance
- **glucocorticoids** (the main endogenous hormones are corticosterone and hydrocortisone (cortisol)) influence carbohydrate and protein metabolism. As well as their metabolic effects they also have anti-inflammatory, anti-allergenic and immunosuppressive actions (Rang et al 1995, Schimmer & George 1998)

A range of synthetic corticosteroids has been developed with the glucocorticoid and mineralocorticoid actions separated. However, it has not been possible to separate the wanted anti-inflammatory actions of the glucocorticoids from their other unwanted side effects (*see* side effects of corticosteroids, p. 22) (Rang et al 1995).

The anti-inflammatory (glucocorticoid) effect of corticosteroid is only advantageous if the mineralocorticoid effect of the drug is low, with little effect on water and electrolyte balance. Prednisolone produces predominantly glucocorticoid effects and is the drug of choice for long-term use by mouth. Cortisone and hydrocortisone are not suitable for long-term use because their mineralocorticoid effects are high, resulting in fluid retention. However, hydrocortisone has less side effects and its moderate anti-inflammatory effect makes it useful for topical application for inflammatory skin conditions and for injection in musculoskeletal intralesional injections. Betamethasone and dexamethasone have insignificant mineralocorticoid effects and high gluco-corticoid effects, making them suitable for administration in high doses where fluid retention is not wanted, e.g. cerebral oedema.

Methylprednisolone and triamcinolone, as glucocorticoids, have anti-inflammatory and immunosuppressive effects but little or no mineralocorticoid effects, making them suitable for musculoskeletal injections.

Glucocorticoids act intracellularly at the target tissue, binding to specific receptor proteins in the nucleus which become activated after interaction with the steroid. The steroid–receptor complex then binds to DNA and either initiates or prevents transcription of certain genes, although the mechanisms by which this modification of gene transcription occurs are not fully understood.

The anti-inflammatory effects of glucocorticoids are thought to occur through decreased generation of prostaglandins. The enzyme cyclo-oxygenase (COX-2) is responsible for producing the prostaglandins involved in inflammation. Exogenous glucocorticoids inhibit COX-2 by inhibiting transcription of the relevant gene, reducing prostaglandin generation in inflammatory cells. There is also evidence that glucocorticoids induce the anti-inflammatory mediator lipocortin (Grillet & Dequeker 1990, Rang et al 1995). Time is required for the changes in gene transcription and protein synthesis, which is clinically significant in that most of the effects of corticosteroids are not immediate, there is generally a delay before the beneficial effects are seen (Schimmer & Parker 1996).

Anti-inflammatory effects of corticosteroid injection

All aspects of the inflammatory response are depressed by corticosteroid, regardless of cause, from the early acute phase of pain, heat, redness and swelling to the later chronic phase in which proliferation and remodelling are affected. Excessive or 'useless' inflammation can benefit greatly from corticosteroid. However, it is generally accepted that corticosteroid is not an appropriate treatment for acute inflammation because of its potent effect on the protective aspects of the inflammatory response, and the delay it causes in fibre formation (Kerlan & Glousman 1989, Nelson et al 1995, Laurence et al 1997).

In the chronic inflammatory phase the balance in collagen synthesis is disrupted and inflammation and proliferation continue side-by-side. Corticosteroid injection can be beneficial in this phase, providing its unwanted effects are recognized, with particular note of the loss of tensile strength in the structure, due to reduced production of collagen and glycosaminoglycans (Stefanich 1986, Grillet & Dequeker 1990, Mazanec 1995, Rang et al 1995). For this reason, relative rest from causative or overuse factors is most important following injection, until the soft tissues are considered to have returned to their functionally normal strength, e.g. approximately 2 weeks following triamcinolone acetonide injection (Cameron 1995a, Drugs and Therapeutic Bulletin 1995, CSP 1999) (see below).

Reduced inflammation and immunosuppression is mainly achieved by the action on blood vessels, inflammatory cells and inflammatory mediators, and involves the following processes (Rang et al 1995, Schimmer and Parker 1996):

- vasoconstriction of small blood vessels
- reduced fluid exudation
- reduced leucocyte infiltration
- reduced production of the inflammatory mediators, prostaglandins, histamine and kinins
- production of anti-inflammatory mediators, lipocortins
- inhibition of the macrophage, delaying phagocytosis, fibroblast activity and ultimately repair
- reduction in the permeability of the synovial membrane; corticosteroid is taken up selectively by the synovium
- reduced migration of leucocytes
- reduced activity of mononuclear cells
- reduced proliferation of blood vessels
- reduced fibrosis

The effect of corticosteroid injection on collagen synthesis in the proliferation and remodelling phases is disputed (Sandberg 1964, Ehrlich & Hunt 1968, Ehrlich et al 1972, Kulick et al 1984). Marks et al (1983) showed a significant delay in wound healing by the application of topical steroids. Long-term, large doses of the sustained-release form of methylprednisolone were found to suppress collagen synthesis, while intermittent doses appeared to have no effect (Cohen et al 1977). Intralesional corticosteroid produces keloid regression by inhibition of fibroblast migration, decreased collagen synthesis and increased collagenase activity (Carrico et al 1984).

In basic terms, an intra-articular or intralesional corticosteroid injection reduces inflammation, alters collagen synthesis and relieves pain. The reduced inflammation and analgesic affect allows the patient to move the affected part more normally. Normal mechanical stress induces collagen fibre orientation and leads to a strong, mobile repair (Stearns 1940a, 1940b, Le Gros Clark 1965, Kesson & Atkins 1998). The altered collagen synthesis may initially weaken collagen fibres and, as a general rule, the patient should be instructed to rest from causative or overusing factors until they are symptom- and sign-free.

Corticosteroids used in musculoskeletal injections

Preparations licensed for intra-articular and intralesional injections (compiled from information contained in manufacturer's data sheets) are listed in Table 3.1. Those highlighted in bold will be used in the examples in the regional section of this book.

Table 3.1 Preparations licensed for intra-articular and intralesional injections

Generic name	Trade name	Dosage	Presentation
Hydrocortisone acetate	Hydrocortistab®	25 mg/ml	1 ml ampoules
Prednisolone acetate	Deltastab®	25 mg/ml	1 ml ampoules
Methylprednisolone acetate	Depo-medrone®*	40 mg/ml	1, 2 & 3 ml vials
Triamcinolone acetonide	**Adcortyl®**	**10 mg/ml**	**1 ml ampoules 5 ml vials**
Triamcinolone acetonide	**Kenalog®**	**40 mg/ml**	**1 ml vials****
Betamethasone sodium phosphate	Betnesol®	4 mg/ml	1 ml ampoules
Dexamethasone sodium phosphate	Organon®	5 mg/ml	2 ml vials and 1 ml ampoules
Dexamethasone sodium phosphate	Decadron®	4 mg/ml***	2 ml vials

* Also available as a combined preparation with lidocaine, containing methylprednisolone 4% and lidocaine 1% in 1 or 2 ml vials; **also available in 1 and 2 ml pre-filled syringes, although these are mainly intended for systemic administration by deep intramuscular injection, rather than intralesional use; *** the quoted dose is actually expressed as the equivalent dose of dexamethasone phosphate.

Relative potency

This is expressed in terms of hydrocortisone as the standard, administered systemically, which is said to have a relative potency of 1. The compartive potencies are listed in Table 3.2.

Table 3.2 Relative potencies of the corticosteroids

Corticosteroid	Relative potency
Hydrocortisone	1
Prednisolone	4
Methylprednisolone	5
Triamcinolone	5
Betamethasone	30
Dexamethasone	30

Duration of action of the corticosteroids

Listed in order, starting with the most relatively soluble and least prolonged, to the least soluble and most prolonged:

- hydrocortisone
- prednisolone acetate
- betamethasone
- dexamethasone
- triamcinolone acetonide
- methylprednisolone acetate

Corticosteroids are categorized according to their duration of action, which varies inversely with the solubility of the drug in water. Preparations such as dexamethasone and betamethasone have relatively more potent anti-inflammatory effects compared to the shorter-acting preparations, such as hydrocortisone, and equivalent doses will therefore vary. For example, 20 mg of hydrocortisone is equivalent to 4 mg of triamcinolone, 5 mg prednisolone and 0.75 mg of dexamethasone (Kerlan & Glousman 1989, Nelson et al 1995, BNF 2000). The medium-acting preparations, such as triamcinolone, fall into the middle range in terms of relative anti-inflammatory potency and equivalent dose.

Hydrocortisone acetate is weak, relatively soluble and is usually absorbed within 36 hours. Synthetic corticosteroids are more potent and less soluble and their anti-inflammatory effects are therefore more prolonged. Precise data on the duration of action is scant, but after peri-articular injection, methylprednisolone acetate remains in the plasma for a mean of 16 days, triamcinolone hexacetonide takes 14–21 days to be absorbed from a joint and triamcinolone acetonide takes slightly less time (Cameron 1995a, Drugs and Therapeutics Bulletin 1995). The duration of action of corticosteroids, once absorbed, is described by the 'plasma half life' of the drug ($t_{1/2}$, i.e. the time taken for the plasma concentration to fall by 50% (*see* Chapter 1).

The corticosteroid used as an example throughout the regional techniques in this book is triamcinolone acetonide (Adcortyl® and Kenalog®, see Figs 3.1 and 3.2). For other drugs and information *see* p. 21 and refer to current manufacturers' data sheets. The recommended dosage given in the regional section is intended as a guideline and is a conservative estimate. It is recommended that the clinician who judges that an injection of corticosteroid is the treatment of choice makes a decision on dosage in line with the guidelines, but also takes into account the severity of the patient's condition, the relative size of the area to be injected and any response to previous injection.

In order to provide immediate pain-relief and to allow confirmation of accurate diagnosis and appropriate treatment, the chosen corticosteroid is injected together with a local anaesthetic agent (Nelson et al 1995, Saunders & Cameron 1997, Kesson & Atkins 1998). Lidocaine is generally the local anaesthetic of choice (*see* p. 27).

Side effects and complications of injected corticosteroids

For contraindications to injections see Chapter 4. Side effects and complications of corticosteroids are generally related to large doses and/or prolonged

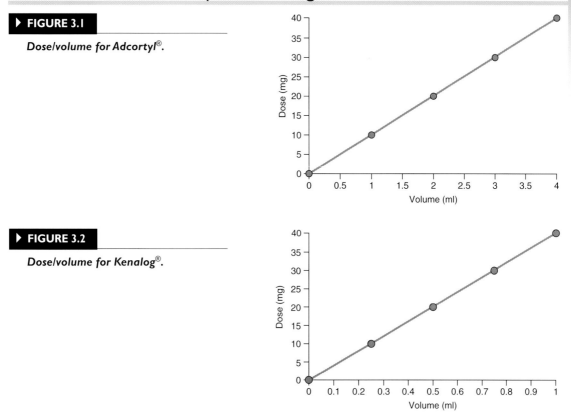

▶ **FIGURE 3.1**

Dose/volume for Adcortyl®.

▶ **FIGURE 3.2**

Dose/volume for Kenalog®.

systemic use. Systemic side effects of a 'one-off' injection of corticosteroid are rare, but can occur. The potential benefits from the prudent use of local corticosteroid injections outweigh their adverse effects (Cooper & Kirwan 1990, Hunter & Blyth 1999). Kumar & Newman (1999) conducted a prospective study to investigate the possible complications associated with intra- and peri-articular steroid injections and found the procedure to be safe with a very low complication rate, if performed while taking adequate precautions. In the section below, the more common side effects associated with local injection of corticosteroid are listed first, followed by the side effects most often associated with systemic use.

Post-injection flare

This is a self-limiting side effect occurring 6–12 hours after injection, once the local anaesthetic effect has worn off, and resolving in less than 72 hours. It is an acute inflammatory reaction considered to be associated with the precipitation of steroid crystals due to the preservatives in the local anaesthetic. The induced synovitis in a joint causes typical symptoms of acute inflammation, i.e. pain, redness, heat and swelling, and similar effects can be induced in a soft tissue injection such as tennis elbow.

A full explanation of the possible side effects should be given and the patient advised to take appropriate measures to reduce the inflammation, such as rest, ice and non-steroidal anti-inflammatory drugs, or simple analgesics.

The symptoms may resemble a septic arthritis and if these symptoms do not abate in the expected time, appropriate action should be taken for this more serious complication (*see* Chapter 2) (Stefanich 1986, Grillet & Dequeker 1990, Mazanec 1995, Swain & Kaplan 1995, Hunter & Blyth 1999).

Local soft tissue atrophy and pigment changes

Fat atrophy (lipotrophy), skin atrophy, senile purpura (small reddish or purple spots occurring under the skin in the elderly) and depigmentation have all been documented. These changes occur more readily with the longer-acting, less soluble drugs such as the triamcinolone preparations and/or through repeated injection into the same site. Causes have also been associated with misplaced injections, i.e. an injection given subcutaneously before the target tissue is reached and/or as a result of leakage of the solution back along the needle track.

The changes are more likely to occur with superficial soft tissue injections such as tennis and golfer's elbow and can appear at the site 6 weeks to 3 months after the injection (Ponec et al 1977, Marks et al 1983, Cooper & Kirwan 1990, Grillet & Dequeker 1990, Pfenninger 1991, Swain & Kaplan 1995). Due to the possible unsightly cosmetic appearance, this potential complication should be discussed with the patient before the injection is performed.

Connective tissue (tendon) weakening

A recognized effect of corticosteroid drugs is a change in the mechanical properties of connective tissue structures, resulting in a loss of tensile strength due to reduced production of collagen and glycosaminoglycans. Following injection, the loss of tensile strength can last for up to 2 weeks and this highlights the importance of specific advice on relative rest following injection.

Tendons in particular have a relatively poor blood supply and are prone to degeneration. Some are notoriously susceptible to rupture, e.g. the Achilles tendon, rotator cuff tendons, the long head of biceps and abductor pollicis longus and extensor pollicis brevis in their shared synovial sheath. It is difficult to find conclusive evidence that corticosteroid injection is directly responsible for tendon rupture, or whether the rupture is in fact due to the degenerative disease process (Kennedy & Baxter Willis 1976, Kleinman & Gross 1983, Mahler & Fritschy 1992, Read & Motto 1992, Speed 2001).

Measures can be taken to minimize the risk of rupture following corticosteroid injection. Advice on relative rest for up to 2 weeks is important. Accurate diagnosis and treatment should avoid the necessity for repeated injections and attention should be paid to the technique itself.

The injection should **never** be delivered directly into the body of the tendon and this is particularly important for weight-bearing tendons and those susceptible to rupture (see above). Bathing the tendon with the corticosteroid solution (*see* Achilles tendon, p. 175) or introducing the solution between a tendon and its sheath (*see* de Quervain's tenosynovitis, p. 102) avoids direct injection into the tendon.

The lesion commonly lies at the teno-osseous junction, where a peppering technique is used. Droplets of corticosteroid solution are delivered at the tendon–bone interface covering the whole area of the lesion and avoiding delivery en masse into one small area (*see* tennis elbow, p. 70).

Notification of tendon damage associated with quinolone antibiotics, e.g. Ciproxin, was delivered from the Committee on Safety of Medicines (CSM 1995). Inflammation and rupture of tendons is a rare complication of this association, but the elderly and those treated concurrently with corticosteroids are considered to be at risk.

Steroid arthropathy

Although steroid arthropathy is a recognized side effect of repeated corticosteroid injections, particularly into weight-bearing joints, the evidence is inconclusive and based mainly on subprimate animal studies (mainly rabbits) and anecdotal case reports. Repeated intra-articular injections are thought to produce a Charcot-type arthropathy with destructive changes in the articular cartilage, although these changes are also seen with the natural progression of the underlying degenerative disease. A Charcot joint is a neurogenic joint where the joint is denervated by some disease process and suffers chronic damage as a result.

Possible mechanisms for the development of steroid arthropathy include joint abuse following corticosteroid-mediated analgesia, with a direct effect on the articular cartilage and ischaemic necrosis (Stefanich 1986, Cooper & Kirwan 1990, Cameron 1995a, Mazanec 1995, Millard & Dillingham 1995). To minimize risk of steroid arthropathy, weight-bearing joints should not be injected more frequently than every 4–6 months.

Iatrogenic (clinician-induced) septic arthritis

This is a rare, but avoidable, complication of corticosteroid injection occurring in 0.001% of patients injected. The organism is typically *Staphylococcus aureus* and the route of infection may be contamination of the injected materials, penetration by skin organisms, haematogenous spread, infection such as respiratory or urogenital tract or a re-activation of a previous infection (Grillet & Dequeker 1990, Haslock et al 1995, Hughes 1996, Coombs & Bax 1996, Hunter & Blyth 1999, Pal & Morris 1999).

The joint becomes red, hot, swollen and painful, but the anti-inflammatory and immunosuppressive properties of the injected corticosteroid may mask the condition and make it difficult to distinguish from a post-injection flare. If symptoms linger after the expected time for post-injection flare (48–72 hours) sepsis should be suspected and treated accordingly. Corticosteroid injection into an already septic joint is absolutely contraindicated, as it will aggravate the condition. If sepsis is suspected, aspiration of a swollen joint should be conducted to eliminate the presence of infection (*see* Chapter 4).

CLINICAL TIP: The complication of septic arthritis can be avoided by screening for current or previous infections, avoiding injection in the presence of skin sepsis and by using a 'no-touch' technique.

Suppression of the response to infection or injury

The anti-inflammatory and immunosuppressive effects of corticosteroids affect the normal response to infection and injury, suppressing clinical signs. Wound healing is also impaired and this would have implications for patients undergoing surgery soon after corticosteroid injection. Steroid warning cards held by patients on long-term corticosteroid therapy include advice on avoiding contact with infectious disease, particularly chickenpox or shingles (BNF 2000).

Facial flushing

Systemic absorption of corticosteroid may cause this benign, transient complication, occurring more readily with triamcinolone preparations in approximately one in 20 patients. Facial flushing can occur within a few minutes of the injection and last for a few hours or up to 1 or 2 days (Neustadt 1991, Nelson et al 1995, BNF 2000).

Menstrual disturbance

With larger injected doses, such as in excess of 40 mg of triamcinolone acetonide, systemic absorption may cause menstrual irregularities and amenorrhoea (ABPI 2000, Saunders and Cameron 1997, Kesson & Atkins 1998).

Hyperglycaemia

Systemic absorption of the injected corticosteroid may produce a transient increase in blood glucose levels in diabetic patients (Mazanec 1995).

Suppression of the hypothalamic–pituitary–adrenal (HPA) axis

Adrenal function is regulated through the HPA axis and suppression of this mechanism reduces the production of endogenous cortisol. Although a more recognized side effect of long-term oral intake of corticosteroids, a single local corticosteroid injection can suppress the HPA axis for 2–4 days (Cooper & Kirwan 1990, Mazanec 1995, Nelson et al 1995, BNF 2000). In long-term corticosteroid therapy, withdrawal should be phased and patients should carry a warning card which indicates that the treatment should not be stopped abruptly.

Iatrogenic Cushing's syndrome

Cushing's syndrome is associated with prolonged use of glucocorticoid therapy, rather than 'one-off' local injections. Alterations occur in fat distribution producing trunk obesity, 'buffalo (dowager's) hump', moon face, muscle wasting and osteoporosis (Cooper & Kirwan 1990, Rang et al 1995).

Osteoporosis

Osteoporosis is a recognized side effect of long-term use of oral corticosteroid therapy and depends on the dosage, duration of the therapy and the disease for which the drugs were prescribed (Cooper & Kirwan 1990, Mazanec 1995). Theoretically, repeated corticosteroid injections could also produce this effect, but this is unlikely to be significant in musculoskeletal injection therapy.

Mood changes

These are more likely to be associated with long-term oral usage, rather than 'one-off' local injections and present typically as euphoria, but may also present as psychosis, agitation, depression and suicidal tendencies. The mood changes are reversible and more likely to occur in patients with pre-existing personality disorders (Cooper & Kirwan 1990, BNF 2000).

Anaphylaxis

Mace et al (1997) document a rare case of anaphylactic shock after an intra-articular injection of synthetic methylprednisolone acetate.

Drug interactions

The following drug interactions have been noted from the ABPI Compendium of Data Sheets and Summaries of Product Characteristics 1999–2000 (ABPI 2000). Corticosteroids:

- antagonize the effect of hypoglycaemic agents including insulin
- antagonize the action of anti-hypertensive agents and diuretics
- enhance the potassium-lowering effect of acetazolamide (Diamox), loop diuretics (e.g. frusemide) and thiazides (e.g. bendrofluazide)

Certain drugs (e.g. barbiturates, carbamazepine, etc.) enhance the metabolic clearance of corticosteroids, but this is not likely to be significant in injection therapy.

LOCAL ANAESTHETICS

Local anaesthetic drugs produce a moderate- to long-lasting, reversible nerve block. With a few exceptions (*see* Carpal tunnel, p. 95) corticosteroid injections are delivered, together with local anaesthetic, in musculoskeletal injections for the following reasons:

- therapeutic pain relief, to allow immediate re-assessment to confirm diagnosis
- to increase the volume effect of the injection in certain conditions, e.g. bursitis

The first known local anaesthetic was cocaine, extracted from coca leaves and used clinically for corneal anaesthesia in 1884, but its toxic effects were found to be excessive. The synthetic substitute procaine was discovered in 1905 and several other compounds were later developed (Rang et al 1995).

Chemically, local anaesthetics consist of an aromatic group linked by an ester or amide bond to a basic side-chain (Rang et al 1995). The ester type, e.g.

procaine, usually comprises generally less stable compounds, while the amide type, e.g. lidocaine and bupivacaine, comprises generally more stable compounds which have a longer plasma half-life.

Mechanism of action

Local anaesthetics penetrate the nerve sheath and axon membrane and block initiation and propagation of the action potential by specifically plugging sodium channels (Rang et al 1995). Conduction is blocked more easily in the small-diameter nerve fibres, producing a reversible local nerve block. Not all fibres are equally susceptible to their action: small, myelinated axons (Aδ fibres) are the most readily blocked, followed by non-myelinated axons (C fibres) and large, myelinated axons (Aβ fibres) are the least readily blocked.

Nociceptive and sympathetic conduction is blocked first. Therefore, pain sensation is blocked more readily than other sensations such as touch and proprioception. Motor axons, which are large in diameter, are relatively resistant to the action of local anaesthetics, but it is difficult to be totally selective to affect pain sensation only and a transient local paralysis may occur.

The potency, toxicity, duration of action, stability and solubility of local anaesthetic drugs vary considerably and those suitable for use in musculoskeletal injections will now be discussed.

Local anaesthetics used in musculoskeletal injections

The local anaesthetics suitable for musculoskeletal injections are listed in Table 3.3.

Table 3.3   Suitable local anaesthetics for musculoskeletal injections

Generic name	Trade name	Dosage	Presentation
Lidocaine hydrochloride 0.5%	Non-proprietary 0.5%*	5 mg/ml	10 ml ampoule
Lidocaine hydrochloride 1%	Non-proprietary 1%*	10 mg/ml	2 ml, 5 ml, 10 ml and 20 ml ampoules
Lidocaine hydrochloride 2%	Non-proprietary 2%*	20 mg/ml	2 ml and 5 ml ampoules
Lidocaine hydrochloride 0.5%	Xylocaine® 0.5%**	5 mg/ml	20 ml vial
Lidocaine hydrochloride 1%	Xylocaine® 1%**	10 mg/ml	20 ml vial
Lidocaine hydrochloride 2%	Xylocaine® 2%**	20 mg/ml	20 ml vial
Bupivacaine hydrochloride 0.25%	Marcain® 0.25%**	2.5 mg/ml	10 ml Polyamp®
Bupivacaine hydrochloride 0.5%	Marcain® 0.5%**	5 mg/ml	10 ml Polyamp®

* BNF 2000; ** ABPI 2000

Relative potency and duration of action

See Table 3.4 for a comparison of lidocaine and bupivacaine.

Table 3.4 Lidocaine and buvipacaine

Lidocaine hydrochloride	Bupivacaine hydrochloride
Rapid rate of onset	Slow rate of onset
Medium duration of action (plasma $t_{1/2}$ of 2 hours)	Long duration of action (plasma $t_{1/2}$ of 3 hours)
Maximum dose 200 mg	Maximum dose 150 mg
Medium potency	Four times as potent as lidocaine (Scott 1989)
Risk: convulsions occur before cardiac arrest and give warning of impending serious toxicity	Risk: irreversible cardiac arrest may occur without preceding convulsions

Maximum doses

The maximum doses recommended in Table 3.4 are for infiltration, not via the intravenous route, and apply to a fit adult of average weight (Scott 1989, BNF 2000). Systemic toxicity is related to blood levels and these vary according to:

- rate at which the drugs are absorbed and excreted
- potency
- patient's age, weight, physique and clinical condition
- degree of vascularity of the area to be injected
- duration of administration

For most regional anaesthetic procedures, maximum arterial plasma concentrations occur within 10–25 minutes, and for this reason patients should be carefully monitored for signs of toxic side effects for up to 30 minutes after administration of local anaesthetics (CSP 1999, BNF 2000).

The maximum safe dose of lidocaine (Fig. 3.3) is possibly higher than the data sheet figure shown, which gives the recognized figures for the UK and Europe. In the USA the recommended maximum dose for lidocaine is 300 mg (Scott 1989, Palve et al 1995).

▶ **FIGURE 3.3**

Dose/volume relationship for local anaesthetic solutions.

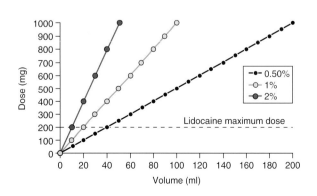

Local anaesthetics combined with adrenaline

Some preparations are combined with adrenaline, which acts as a vaso-constrictor diminishing blood plasma levels and permitting a higher dose of local anaesthetic to be given (Scott 1989, BNF 2000). Although the effect of the local anaesthetic will be prolonged, possible additional complications include potential ischaemic damage, and the combined use of local anaesthetics with adrenaline is absolutely contraindicated in the digits. Susceptibility to cardiac arrhythmias may also be increased. Local anaesthetic combined with adrenaline is **not** recommended for musculoskeletal injections (CSP 1999).

Side effects and complications of injected local anaesthetics

Adhering to the maximum recommended doses (see above) should avoid serious side effects and complications of local anaesthetic drugs. For contra-indications to injections see Chapter 4. Inadvertent intravenous injection is most likely to cause problems, and for this reason it is recommended that once the needle is judged to be within the target tissue, aspiration is conducted to ensure that there is no flow-back of blood indicating placement within a blood vessel.

Central nervous system toxicity tends to occur more readily with the ester-type local anaesthetics, e.g. procaine, than with the amide-type, e.g. lidocaine and bupivacaine (Rang et al 1995, BNF 2000).

Central nervous system effects

Local anaesthetics initially cause stimulation of the central nervous system, which may be perceived as:

- a feeling of inebriation and light headedness
- restlessness and tremor
- confusion
- extreme agitation

Further increase of the drug leads to depression of the central nervous system, which may be perceived as:

- sedation
- twitching
- convulsions
- respiratory depression which is potentially life-threatening

CLINICAL TIP: Procaine is rarely used now as it provides less intense analgesia because of its reduced spread through the tissues (BNF 2000). It has been replaced by lidocaine as the local anaesthetic of choice for musculoskeletal injections.

Cardiovascular effects

These are mainly:

- Myocardial depression (due to the blocking of sodium channels in the cardiac muscle reducing calcium stores and, in turn, reducing myocardial contraction) could potentially lead to cardiac arrest. However, lidocaine is useful, in the appropriate clinical setting, for its role in the treatment of arrhythmias.
- Vasodilatation is due partly to the drug's effect on the vascular smooth muscle and partly to sympathetic inhibition.
- Hypotension, as a result of myocardial depression and vasodilatation, can be sudden and life-threatening.

Allergic reactions

These are covered in greater detail in Chapter 2. The most common is an allergic dermatitis due to hypersensitivity. Rarely, an acute anaphylactic reaction can occur which is life-threatening.

Drug interactions

Cimetidine (Tagamet®), an anti-ulcer drug, may delay the metabolism of lidocaine, but this is probably of little significance with the doses advocated (ABPI 2000). A metabolite of procaine (para amino benzoic acid) inhibits the action of sulphonamide antibiotics, but this is not relevant in this text since musculoskeletal injections in the presence of infection are contraindicated (Rang et al 1995).

CONCLUSION

This chapter has given an overview of the principal drugs used in musculo-skeletal injections, with notes on their mechanism of action, effects, side-effects and possible complications. The following chapter will provide general injection principles and will complete the theory section that underpins the application of injection therapy.

4 General injection principles

CHAPTER SUMMARY

This chapter provides the general principles of injection therapy by firstly addressing the absolute and relative contraindications for the administration of injections. A discussion of general and specific techniques follows, with a guidance for a 'no-touch' technique and notes on follow up management and advice to be given to the patient to enhance effectiveness. Key points of record-keeping are listed and a suggested treatment regime is presented. A flow chart for the clinical decision-making process towards the administration of an injection concludes the section.

CONTRAINDICATIONS

The reader is referred to the *Clinical Guideline for the Use of Injection Therapy by Physiotherapists* (CSP 1999), which provides evidence for absolute and relative contraindications to musculoskeletal injections.

Absolute contraindications are:

- infection in the joint
- local sepsis or any infective illness
- hypersensitivity/allergy to steroid or local anaesthetic
- adjacent osteomyelitis

Relative contraindications to musculoskeletal injection are:

- recent history of trauma
- anticoagulant therapy
- bleeding disorders
- poorly controlled diabetes
- prosthetic joint
- haemarthrosis

- psychogenic or anxious patient
- concurrent oral corticosteroid therapy

The following should also be considered cautiously:

- pregnancy, especially in the first trimester (Silver 1999), but the final risk–benefit decision should be left to the medical practitioner
- recent history of malignancy
- children and adolescents; may have an effect on skeletal growth and maturity (CSP 1999, Nelson et al 1995)

Musculoskeletal injections should only be delivered following a full assessment of the patient, taking into account the history (subjective examination) and examination (objective examination) which lead to clinical diagnosis. Hollingworth et al (1983), in a randomized, double-blind study, concluded that the anatomical method of injection after diagnosis by selective tension was more successful than using trigger- or tender-point location. Jones et al (1993) studied the accuracy of placement of joint injections and found surprisingly poor accuracy of delivery, particularly at the knee and shoulder, the two most commonly injected joints. Haslock et al (1995), in a questionnaire to 172 consultant rheumatologists, found that there was no single consensus technique for intra-articular and soft tissue injections.

The term 'selective tension' was originally introduced by Cyriax and describes the process of using passive movements to test the inert structures, and resisted movements to test the contractile structures (Cyriax & Cyriax 1983, Cyriax 1984). The logical method of subjective and objective examination which, by reasoned elimination, leads to the incrimination of the affected tissue and the specific site of the lesion, is described fully in the companion text *Orthopaedic Medicine: a Practical Approach* (Kesson & Atkins 1998).

If injection is judged to be the treatment of choice, the procedure, including benefits and risks, should be fully explained to the patient in order to obtain informed consent. The wishes of a patient to decline injection should be respected. The legal age for consent is 16.

At the time of writing, physiotherapists do not have prescribing rights under the terms of the Medicines Act 1968. However, as a step in that direction, group protocols have been put into place in some areas that allow physiotherapists to administer named drugs to patients without obtaining individual prescriptions from medical practitioners. In all other circumstances, injection by physiotherapists should be with the agreement of the patient's medical practitioner, who is responsible for prescribing the injectable drugs, but the physiotherapist remains responsible for administering the injection (CSP 1999).

The equipment required for injection should be assembled and checked. The area to be injected should be prepared, taking into account the precise location of the target tissue, route of access to the lesion, avoidance of vulnerable structures such as nerves and blood vessels, and patient and operator comfort. The choice of needle will depend on the location and size of the target tissue, but in general terms, this should be the finest needle that will reach the full extent of the lesion. The choice of syringe will depend on the volume of the injection to be delivered.

The dose to be administered will depend on the nature and size of the lesion, the severity of the condition and any response to previous injections. The reader is recommended to use the example doses from the regional section, which are intended as a guide, and which for safety tend towards the conservative.

Using triamcinolone acetonide as an example of an injectable corticosteroid, dosage would be Adcortyl® 10 mg/ml or Kenalog® 40 mg/ml, with lidocaine 1% as an example local anaesthetic (see Table 4.1).

Table 4.1   Dosage example for different applications

Structure	Corticosteroid dose	Corticosteroid volume	Local anaesthetic volume	Total volume
Small tendons, e.g. tennis elbow	10 mg	0.25 ml Kenalog®	0.75 ml 1% lidocaine	1 ml
Large tendons, e.g. adductor longus	20 mg	0.5 ml Kenalog®	1 ml 1% lidocaine	1.5 ml
Small joints, e.g. acriomioclavicular	5–10 mg	0.25 ml Kenalog®	0.25 ml 1% lidocaine	0.5 ml
Large joints, e.g. hip	Up to 40 mg	4 ml Adcortyl®	1 ml 1% lidocaine	5 ml

'NO-TOUCH' TECHNIQUE FOR MUSCULOSKELETAL INJECTIONS

The following guidance for a no-touch technique is suggested to minimize the risk of infection.

- Note any previous allergic reaction to injections, since this will contra-indicate continuing with the procedure.
- Check the drugs to be used, choose an appropriate-sized needle and syringe. Note the expiry dates on the containers, needles and syringes.
- Consider the precise location of the anatomical structure to be injected and the possible route of access to the lesion. Position the patient with the lesion and injection site accessible, bearing in mind patient comfort and that of the operator.
- Mark the injection site, e.g. with the end of the needle sheath, retracted end of a ballpoint pen, fingernail or skin marker pen.
- Wash and dry hands preferably with surgical scrub or antiseptic soap.
- Clean the skin over the injection site with a suitable antiseptic, e.g. chlor-hexidine 0.5% in spirit or Mediswab™ (Cawley & Morris 1992). Draw up the drug using single-dose containers wherever possible.
- Disposable needles are inexpensive, therefore change the needle after draw-ing up the drug, in case of contamination.
- Deliver the injection using a 'no-touch' technique. Neither the prepared injection site nor the needle should be touched. If withdrawing the needle to change to a different entry site, the needle should again be changed before the second insertion (e.g. injection of the Achilles tendon, p. 175).
- Once the needle is judged to be within the target tissue, aspiration should be carried out to ensure that it is not placed within a blood vessel, before the injection is delivered.

- Withdraw the needle and dispose of it and the syringe safely (*see* Chapter 2).
- Apply pressure over the puncture site using cotton wool.
- Apply a suitable dressing, e.g. sticking plaster, having ensured that the patient is not allergic to such materials.

An accurate knowledge of anatomy is vital. Needle entry should be made quickly through the skin, using appropriate anatomical landmarks and guidelines to aim towards the target tissue (*see* Section 2).

The sensation of resistance imparted as the needle passes through the different tissues varies and allows the clinician to judge where the needle is placed. Injections should never be given directly into the body of a tendon, which will be felt as a fairly solid resistance. At the teno-osseous junction, where the solution is delivered at the bone–tendon interface, the bony sensation will be appreciated. It is important to be gentle as the needle point contacts bone, as this can be painful for the patient. Injection into a tendon sheath (tenosynovitis) should have a sensation of little or no resistance and the sheath may be seen to fill and swell slightly. Injection into a joint capsule or bursa will be experienced as a loss of resistance to the needle, indicating placement in a space. The patient may be aware of the needle reaching the target tissue and report a provocation of their symptoms. For nerve entrapment syndromes (e.g. carpal tunnel) the solution is delivered to bathe the inflamed nerve. Any reports of paraesthesia indicate that the needle is in the nerve and must be immediately withdrawn.

Once the needle is judged to be in the target tissue, the plunger should be drawn back slightly to check that placement is not within a blood vessel. If there is a back-flow of blood, the needle should be withdrawn and firm pressure applied to the area, before repositioning the needle and checking again before injecting.

A joint injection should be checked for the presence of infection. Once in situ, the plunger should be drawn back slightly and the fluid drawn into the syringe inspected. If this is a clear, straw-coloured solution it is normal, and the injection can proceed. If the withdrawn fluid is opalescent or cloudy, this indicates possible infection and the injection of corticosteroid should not proceed. Medical practitioners may wish to aspirate the joint and send the fluid for culture. Physiotherapists should refer the patient back to the medical practitioner, but guidelines for aspiration are under development.

INJECTION TECHNIQUES

Accurate delivery to the target tissue is important to prevent soft tissue changes and subcutaneous leakage. The technique used to deliver the injection will depend on the structure.

Peppering technique

This is a technique used to inject at the teno-osseous junction. The aim is to deliver small droplets of corticosteroid solution over the whole extent of the lesion. These are delivered at the tendon–bone junction. The hard sensation of bone is experienced and the needle is withdrawn very slightly from the bone to deliver each droplet. This ensures that the droplets of solution are evenly distributed throughout the lesion, rather than a concentrated bolus at one location. The body of the tendon itself should not be injected.

Bolus technique

This technique is used to inject bursae, joints, tendon sheaths and other areas such as the carpal tunnel. The aim is to deliver the corticosteroid solution as a whole, with one continuous squeeze of the plunger, into the bursal or joint space, where there should be no resistance to the injection.

SUBSEQUENT MANAGEMENT

Once the injection has been delivered, the patient may rest for a few minutes before the positive objective findings are re-assessed. The use of local anaesthetic should temporarily abolish symptoms, which allows the clinician to check diagnosis and accurate needle placement. Ideally, the patient should be kept under further observation for up to 30 minutes after the injection to monitor for any adverse reaction, particularly anaphylaxis (*see* Chapter 3) (CSP 1999, BNF 2000).

The patient should be instructed in the self-management of their condition. Relative rest from causative and aggravating factors is advised for up to 2 weeks following the injection. The injection may form part of a rehabilitation programme and appropriate physiotherapy may be required once the injection has had its effects. The cause of overuse lesions must be established to prevent recurrence.

The patient should be reviewed between 1 and 2 weeks after the injection. The injection can be repeated if the patient is partially improved, but not if the first injection failed to benefit the condition. It is recommended that no more than two corticosteroid injections be given into one structure per annum, except for the glenohumeral joint where a maximum of three injections may be necessary for the treatment of traumatic arthritis (frozen shoulder). Due to the risk of steroid arthropathy (*see* Chapter 3), weight-bearing joints should not be injected more frequently than every 4–6 months.

As mentioned previously in Chapter 3, it is important to highlight the recommendation that if two structures require injection in one treatment session, the total dose of corticosteroid should not exceed 60 mg of triamcinolone acetonide (or the equivalent for other corticosteroid drugs). If a dose exceeding 40 mg of steroid is given, it may be advisable to issue a steroid card to the patient. In order to keep within the safety margins for local anaesthetic, it is recommended that no more than 5 ml of 1% lidocaine or 15 ml of 0.5% lidocaine should be given on one occasion. These figures are well below the maximum recommended doses and deliberately err on the side of caution, while permitting effective treatment.

RECORD-KEEPING

Detailed clinical records should always be maintained, whatever the treatment of choice for the patient. When considering the use of a musculoskeletal injection, questions relating to the following need particular consideration:

- details of current medications, particularly anticoagulants, insulin or oral diabetic medication
- any significant medical conditions which may contraindicate the injection, produce specific side effects or lead to the possibility of drug interactions
- past allergic reactions, particularly those relating to corticosteroids, local anaesthetics (e.g. following dental procedures) or sticking plaster
- past history of previous problems with joint or soft tissue injections.
- recent or recurrent infections e.g. tuberculosis

The injection site should be examined for evidence of local infection, e.g. boils. Any such infection should be noted in the records and would constitute a contraindication to injection.

The details of the drugs used should be noted:

- prescribing medical practitioner
- name of the drug
- strength of the solution if relevant (e.g. lidocaine 0.5% or 1%)
- dose given
- manufacturer
- batch number
- expiry date

The last three items will be relevant if problems arise from a defective preparation, in which case the manufacturer will be liable. Without this information, liability remains with the prescriber and injector.

Any post-injection advice to the patient should be noted and the date for follow-up recorded. At the follow-up appointment, findings on re-assessment should be noted, in particular any adverse reaction reported or observed should be recorded and physiotherapists should inform the patient's medical practitioner.

SUGGESTED TREATMENT REGIME

The general principles to be applied in the application of injection therapy are summarized in the following suggested treatment regime:

1. Take a full history and perform a physical examination of the patient, to reach a clinical diagnosis and be able to formulate a treatment plan.
2. Discuss the possible alternative treatment choices with the patient.
3. Explain the procedure fully to the patient, including any risk, and obtain informed consent (CSP 1999, Gilberthorpe 1996). Allow the patient time to consider the injection so that consent can be freely given; the legal age for consent is 16.
4. If injection is the treatment of choice, the physiotherapist should liaise with the patient's medical practitioner to discuss the prescription for the

drugs (at the time of writing the introduction of prescription rights for physiotherapists is under discussion).

5. Prepare for the injection procedure, with strict adherence to the no-touch technique described above (p. 34).

6. Deliver the injection.

7. Re-assess the patient where appropriate, approximately 5 minutes after the injection, using the positive findings on examination to assess the successful placement of the injection.

8. Give advice on suitable relative rest and rehabilitation.

9. It is recommended that the patient should be asked to remain at the surgery/practice for 30 minutes following the injection (*see* Chapter 3, p. 29).

10. Make a follow-up appointment.

11. Complete the patient's medical records.

CONCLUSION

This chapter has concluded Section 1 by presenting an overview of the general principles of administering musculoskeletal injections. Rifat & Moeller (2001) suggest that joint and soft tissue injection procedures are relatively easy to master, once an understanding of the techniques and subtleties of performing these procedures at certain sites have been acquired. Guidance for a 'no-touch' technique has been included to minimize the risk of infection, and the key points of record-keeping and a suggested treatment regime draw the principles for the application of an injection together.

The clinical decision-making process to be applied in making the decision to inject is presented as a flow chart (Fig. 4.1), which guides the operator by steps through to the administration of the injection, and beyond to the advice on management to be given to the patient and the subsequent re-assessment of treatment outcomes.

Section 2, following, will provide information and suggestions for the application of specific injection techniques and will build on the theory developed within this and the preceding chapters.

▶ **FIGURE 4.1**

The clinical decision-making process.

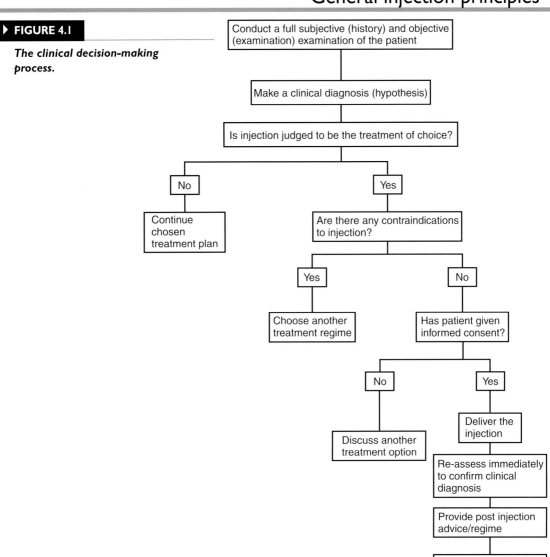

Conduct a full subjective (history) and objective (examination) examination of the patient

Make a clinical diagnosis (hypothesis)

Is injection judged to be the treatment of choice?

No — Continue chosen treatment plan

Yes — Are there any contraindications to injection?

Yes — Choose another treatment regime

No — Has patient given informed consent?

No — Discuss another treatment option

Yes — Deliver the injection

Re-assess immediately to confirm clinical diagnosis

Provide post injection advice/regime

Arrange follow up assessment

2 Practice of musculoskeletal injections – regional injection techniques

Introduction to Section 2

This section presents intra-articular and intralesional injection techniques for peripheral musculoskeletal lesions encountered within clinical practice. The techniques presented have been developed from the original work of Cyriax (Cyriax & Cyriax 1983, Cyriax 1984) and are considered to be in common practice in sports and orthopaedic medicine. A regional approach is adopted, with the injections being categorized into those of the shoulder, elbow, wrist and hand, hip, knee and the ankle and foot.

For clarity, each of the injections described will be presented in a consistent format detailing indications, presentation, needle size, dosage, patient position, palpation of the site, technique of the injection and aftercare advice for the patient. The injection dosages are given as guidelines throughout, and the reader is encouraged to adapt and develop those suggested on the basis of clinical experience. Preparation of the skin for injection and the guidance suggested for a 'no-touch' technique can be found in Section 1, Chapter 4.

Patient presentation of the various conditions is detailed according to an examination procedure using selective tension, devised by Cyriax (Cyriax & Cyriax 1983, Cyriax 1984, Kesson & Atkins 1998). Lesions are described as capsular (in which the specific range of limited movement indicates an arthritis in the joint), non-capsular (which may indicate a bursitis or ligamentous lesion) or contractile (indicating tendinitis or muscle belly lesion where pain is reproduced on the appropriate resisted testing).

Throughout this section, triamcinolone acetonide is used as an example of an injectable steroid, but an equivalent dose of any other corticosteroid preparation may be substituted. The longer-acting corticosteroid preparations have relatively more potent anti-inflammatory properties compared to the shorter-acting preparations, and for this reason equivalent doses will vary, e.g. 4 mg triamcinolone is equivalent to 20 mg hydrocortisone, 5 mg prednisolone and 0.75 mg of dexamethasone. See Chapter 3, or refer to the relevant manufacturer's data sheet for further information (Kerlan & Glousman 1989, Nelson et al 1995, BNF 2000).

Accuracy in the initial diagnosis and in needle placement is paramount and the tips for palpation and technique aim to facilitate and ensure the effectiveness of the injection.

5 The shoulder

GLENOHUMERAL JOINT

Indication

Capsulitis or 'frozen shoulder', which may present as either primary or secondary frozen shoulder. Primary or idiopathic frozen shoulder is sometimes known as steroid-sensitive or monarticular rheumatoid arthritis (Cyriax & Cyriax 1983, Cyriax 1984) and occurs without obvious causative trauma. The more common secondary frozen shoulder may be a progression from traumatic arthritis, or may be associated with other lesions including cervical spine disorders, thoracic immobility, surgery, neurological disease or systemic disease such as diabetes mellitus (Anton 1993, Grubbs 1993, Stam 1994). Changes in anatomical structures closely related to the glenohumeral joint, e.g. the subacromial bursa, rotator cuff tendons or the long head of biceps, may have a secondary effect on the joint capsule (Kesson & Atkins 1998).

Patient presentation

The patient describes pain, gradually increasing over several weeks, which is usually felt in the deltoid region but may refer further into the area of the C5 dermatome (the anterolateral aspect of the arm and forearm as far as the base of the thumb), depending on the irritability of the condition. There is stiffness and loss of functional movement, and the patient may be unable to sleep on the affected side, also indicating a high level of irritability.

On examination, passive movements are limited in the capsular pattern, with a greater proportional loss of lateral rotation, less limitation of abduction and least limitation of medial rotation. The loss of medial rotation has the most functional significance for the patient and restricts such activities as reaching into the back pocket or doing up the bra. The overall limitation of passive movements reduces the range of active elevation and the restricted movements have an abnormal hard end-feel.

Treatment by injection

The aim of corticosteroid injection is to relieve inflammation and pain, allowing the range of functional movement to be restored. Cyriax and Cyriax (1983) and Cyriax (1984) suggested a course of corticosteroid injections given over increasing intervals. As a general rule one, two or a maximum of three injections may be needed for the symptoms to fully subside, depending on the irritability of the condition at assessment. Typical time intervals would be 10–14 days between the first and second injections and 3–4 weeks between the second and third, aiming to give the follow-up injection before the effect of the previous one has completely worn off.

Van der Windt et al (1998) and Dacre et al (1989) both demonstrate the beneficial effects of corticosteroid injections for the treatment of painful stiff shoulders although conversely, in a systematic review of the literature, Van der Heijden et al (1996) found scarce evidence in favour of the efficacy of corticosteroid injections for shoulder lesions, considering the methods of most studies to be of poor quality.

Cameron (1995b) suggested that injections of corticosteroid are efficacious in treating frozen shoulder, providing the patients selected fulfil the diagnostic criteria based on the Cyriax assessment and the patient presentation summarized above (for more detail see Kesson & Atkins 1998).

Needle size	21 G × $1^1/_2$ in (0.8 × 40 mm) or 2 in (0.8 × 50 mm) green needle.

Dose	20–30 mg triamcinolone acetonide, 1 ml local anaesthetic, e.g. 2–3 ml Adcortyl®, 1 ml 1% lidocaine.
	The evidence suggests that the corticosteroid is the most important component of the injection (Jacobs et al 1991). Some authorities advocate the use of much larger volumes of local anaesthetic to cause distension of the joint capsule (Gam et al 1998). De Jong et al (1998) conducted a comparative study which showed that in the treatment of frozen shoulder greater symptom relief was gained in a group of patients receiving 40 mg of triamcinolone acetonide, compared with a group receiving 10 mg.

Patient position

Place the patient sitting or in prone lying. A posterior approach is recommended. Rest the arm with the elbow in flexion across the front of the waist to position the shoulder into medial rotation, so opening out the posterior aspect of the joint.

Palpation

Stand behind the patient and place the thumb of your non-injecting hand on the posterior angle of the acromion, with your index or middle finger placed anteriorly on the coracoid process. Mark a point approximately 1 cm below your thumb.

Technique

Insert the needle at the marked point and direct the needle forward, aiming towards your finger placed on the coracoid process (Fig. 5.1). Proceed steadily through the different tissue layers and once you have felt either the needle piercing the slightly tougher joint capsule, or coming to rest against the 'sticky' articular surface of the humerus, deliver the injection as a bolus (Fig. 5.2). If resistance is felt as the plunger is pressed, the needle tip may be within the articular cartilage. Withdraw slightly and continue with the injection.

CLINICAL TIP: Note that the suprascapular artery and nerve pass through the suprascapular notch and posteriorly around the neck of the scapula. Avoid injecting into these structures by ensuring accuracy in palpation and the angle of needle entry.

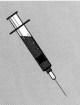

ALTERNATIVE TECHNIQUE: An anterior approach can be used. Position the patient in sitting or lying and palpate the coracoid process. Insert the needle below and lateral to the coracoid process aiming towards the glenohumeral joint. Deliver by a bolus technique when there is no resistance to the injection.

CLINICAL TIP: Note that the axillary artery and brachial plexus lie medial to the coracoid process, deep to pectoralis minor, and the cephalic vein passes between the antero-medial border of deltoid and pectoralis major

Patient advice

The patient should be instructed to begin gentle mobilization as early as pain relief allows. Injection, together with physiotherapeutic advice on an appropriate exercise regime to include scapular stabilization and normal movement patterns, is helpful. The loss of movement in the capsular pattern prevents normal scapulothoracic rhythm with the scapula moving abnormally early during glenohumeral movement.

▶ **FIGURE 5.1**

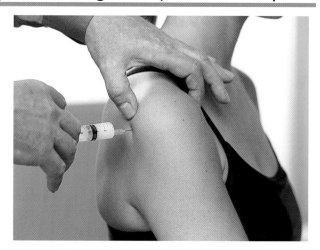

▶ **FIGURE 5.2**

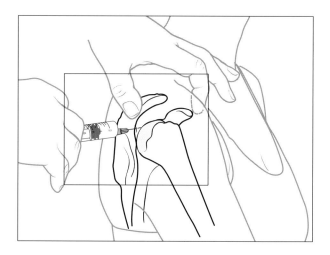

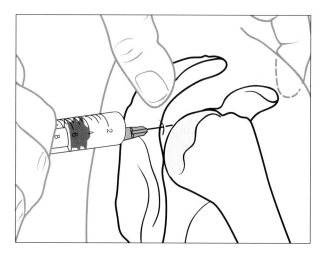

SUBACROMIAL BURSA (SUBDELTOID BURSA)

Indication

Chronic subacromial bursitis and acute subacromial bursitis. Chronic subacromial bursitis is an extremely common cause of pain at the shoulder, but it may present a challenge to diagnosis through the muddled picture presented on examination (Kesson & Atkins 1998). The close anatomical relationship this bursa has with surrounding structures means that it is common for lesions such as bursitis, tendinitis and capsulitis to co-exist at the shoulder. Congenital abnormalities of the acromion or degenerative changes in the acromio-clavicular joint may reduce the subacromial space and surgery may be an option if the bursitis is resistant to treatment.

Acute subacromial bursitis is a completely separate entity from the common chronic subacromial bursitis and has a characteristic onset, which is described below.

Patient presentation

Chronic subacromial bursitis is generally due to repeated impingement of the bursa. The patient complains of a gradual onset of low-grade aching over the deltoid area, with increased pain on reaching movements with the arm at shoulder height, such as putting on a coat or car seat-belt. They may have trouble sleeping on that side and may find pushing down through the arm painful, since this action increases impingement of the bursa under the coraco-acromial arch.

On examination, a non-capsular pattern with a full range of active and passive movement is usually present. Full passive elevation may increase the symptoms, but the normal elastic end-feel exists. A painful arc may be present on active abduction, indicating impingement of the inflamed bursa under the acromion. The application, or release, of resisted tests may compress the bursa and produce symptoms, hence the 'muddle' of signs mentioned above. A similar pattern of signs may be found with rotator cuff lesions, especially if more than one tendon is involved, for example, both supraspinatus and infraspinatus.

Acute subacromial bursitis is a rarer condition and typically presents with a rapid onset of severe pain over several hours, the pain gradually referring through the extent of the C5 dermatome (the antero-lateral aspect of the arm and forearm as far as the base of the thumb). Sleep is disturbed by the acute nature of the pain, leaving the patient looking tired and unwell. Voluntary muscle spasm ensures that the patient holds the arm in an antalgic (pain-avoiding) posture to avoid the severe twinges of pain that are experienced on active movement. Acute subacromial bursitis has a similar presentation to acute calcific tendinitis and it may be debated that both terms are describing the same underlying condition.

On examination the patient will tolerate very little movement, particularly towards abduction. The condition is usually self-limiting, with the severe pain decreasing in approximately 7–10 days, but the condition may not settle completely for up to 6 weeks.

Treatment by injection

The treatment for chronic subacromial bursitis is an injection of a large volume of low-dose local anaesthetic with an appropriate amount of cortico-steroid. However, this is unlikely to have a lasting effect in itself, unless the mechanisms by which the bursa becomes inflamed are addressed (see below).

In acute subacromial bursitis a smaller overall volume of fluid is delivered to the already swollen bursa. This may initially increase the symptoms before the anti-inflammatory effects of the corticosteroid lead to a reduction in the pain.

Needle size	21 G × 1$\frac{1}{2}$ in (0.8 × 40 mm) green needle.

Dose	**Chronic subacromial bursitis**
	20 mg triamcinolone acetonide, 5 ml local anaesthetic, e.g. 2 ml Adcortyl®, 5 ml 0.5% or 1% lidocaine.
	Acute subacromial bursitis
	20 mg triamcinolone acetonide, 1 ml local anaesthetic, e.g. 2 ml Adcortyl®, 1 ml 1% lidocaine.

Patient position

Seat the patient with the arm resting pendant by the side.

Palpation

Palpate the lateral border of the acromion to locate the groove between the acromion and head of the humerus. The subacromial bursa caps the greater tuberosity and extends under the acromion as far as the acromioclavicular joint line. It is this subacromial portion of the bursa that you aim to inject. Mark a point approximately at the mid-point of the acromion.

Technique

Insert the needle just below the mid-point of the acromion, angling it slightly upwards until it lies between the acromion and head of the humerus (Fig. 5.3). Deliver the injection as a bolus when a loss of resistance is identified (Fig. 5.4). In chronic bursitis, synovial folds and adhesions may prevent this bolus delivery and it may be necessary to deliver the injection by a horizontal

▶ FIGURE 5.3

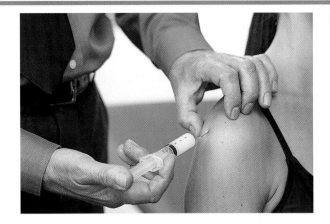

▶ FIGURE 5.4

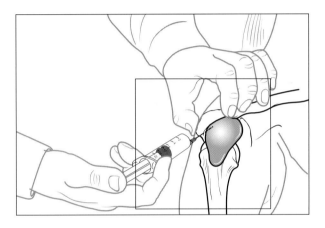

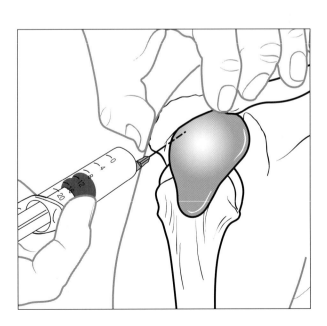

peppering technique. Reproduction of the patient's pain as you inject is usually an indication of accuracy of positioning of the injection.

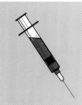

ALTERNATIVE TECHNIQUE:
1. A posterior approach: the needle is inserted just below the posterior angle of the acromion (the posterior 'eye' of the shoulder in acupuncture) and angled forward.
2. An anterior approach: the needle is inserted under the anterior edge of the acromion, lateral to the acriomioclavicular joint.

Patient advice

After the injection for either the chronic or acute conditions, the patient should be advised to rest from overuse activities. In the case of chronic subacromial bursitis, the cause of impingement should be identified. The restoration of normal muscle balance forces around the shoulder is important to normal movement and prevents excessive superior translation of the humerus, which is a key factor in the development of 'impingement syndrome'.

ACROMIOCLAVICULAR JOINT

Indication

Arthritis due to overuse or degeneration of the acromioclavicular joint, or strain following trauma.

Patient presentation

The patient complains of pain specifically localized to the acromioclavicular joint at the point of the shoulder. Usually the patient points to the pain with a single finger rather than using the whole hand.

On examination of the glenohumeral joint, there is a non-capsular pattern of movement with pain felt at the end of range of all passive movements, i.e. passive elevation and medial and lateral rotation. Diagnosis is confirmed by a positive 'scarf test', i.e. pain on combined passive horizontal flexion and adduction.

Treatment by injection

Injection may be successful in minor sprains of the acromioclavicular joint or arthritis (Jacob & Sallay 1997). Dislocation or recurrent subluxation of the joint may require surgical intervention.

Needle size	23 G × 1 in (0.6 × 25 mm) blue needle or 25 G × ⁵/₈ in (0.5 × 16 mm) orange needle.

Dose	10 mg triamcinolone acetonide, 0.25 ml local anaesthetic, e.g. 0.25 mg Kenalog®, 0.25 ml 1% lidocaine.

Patient position

Place the patient in sitting or half lying.

Palpation

Palpate for the superior aspect of the acromioclavicular joint line, which will lie approximately 1–2 cm medial to the lateral border of the acromion. The clavicle tends to override the acromion and a bump or step may be felt. Gentle superior/inferior movement of the clavicle may aid the localization of the joint line.

Technique

Insert the needle, angled inferiorly and slightly medially, through the superior capsular ligament, and once in the joint deliver the injection as a bolus (Figs 5.5 and 5.6).

CLINICAL TIP: This joint can be difficult to inject because it may be narrowed due to degenerative changes and surrounding osteophytes. An articular disc dropping down into the joint space from the superior capsular ligament can also impede entry. Skill may be required in 'palpating' for the joint space with the needle, involving consideration for the angle of entry. The superior ligament can be injected using a peppering technique if entry into the joint is not possible.

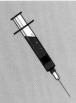

ALTERNATIVE TECHNIQUE: An anterior approach can be used where the needle is inserted into the anterior 'v-shaped' notch between the clavicle and acromion, aiming backwards, in a horizontal line with the joint surfaces.

Patient advice

Advise the patient to maintain a period of relative rest for up to 2 weeks after the injection.

▶ **FIGURE 5.5**

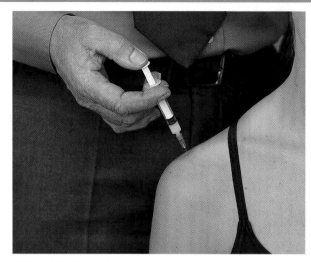

▶ **FIGURE 5.6**

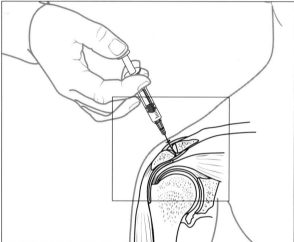

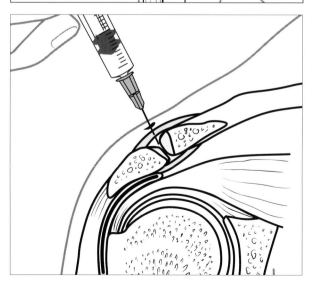

ROTATOR CUFF TENDONS

Indication

Contractile lesion at the shoulder, which may involve one of the rotator cuff tendons of supraspinatus, infraspinatus or subscapularis. The lesion can vary from simple strain to degeneration involving full- or partial-thickness tears. The cause is usually overuse resulting in cumulative microtrauma of the tendon. Fatigue and degeneration may then result in muscle imbalance and abnormal movement patterns. The head of the humerus is no longer effectively depressed by the action of the rotator cuff muscles, resulting in abnormal superior translation and further trauma to the tendons through impingement.

Patient presentation

The patient describes pain of gradual onset with single traumatic incidents being possible, but less common. Pain is felt over the deltoid area of the shoulder and is increased by activity, particularly involving the use of the hands above shoulder level. Chronic, long-term lesions can lead to involvement of the other closely related anatomical structures, i.e. the subacromial bursa and/or the joint capsule.

On examination, an uncomplicated tendinitis presents with pain on the appropriate resisted test and possibly pain on the opposite passive movement. However, the principal signs are:

- supraspinatus: pain on resisted abduction
- infraspinatus: pain on resisted lateral rotation
- subscapularis: pain on resisted medial rotation

Localizing signs may exist which help to locate the exact site of the lesion. In the case of supraspinatus and infraspinatus, the presence of a painful arc incriminates the teno-osseous junction of the tendon. In subscapularis, a painful arc incriminates the upper fibres, and a positive 'scarf' test (combined passive horizontal flexion and adduction of the shoulder joint) incriminates the lower fibres. Ultimately, palpation of the identified structure will reveal the exact site of the lesion.

Treatment by injection

Injection of simple tendinitis can be curative, provided that the exact site of the lesion is located. Establishing and eliminating the cause of the problem is also important. Complicated cases can be more resistant to treatment, especially if partial- or full-thickness tears exist, and the patient may require surgical investigation. Ultrasound scanning can be useful in identifying the exact pathology present. More chronic lesions may lead to secondary capsulitis, in which case the joint itself may require injection as described for capsulitis or 'frozen shoulder', above.

CLINICAL TIP: Some authorities disagree with injecting individual rotator cuff tendons. Degenerative tears of these tendons are relatively common and there are some reported cases of tendon rupture following corticosteroid injection (see Kesson & Atkins 1998, Chapter 3). An 'umbrella' injection under the acromion may effectively bathe these lesions, as described for the injection of subacromial bursitis (p. 47).

Injection of the rotator cuff tendons is just one treatment option and another is transverse friction massage by a physiotherapist. Whatever the choice of treatment, the cause of the overuse activity and/or reason for impingement must be addressed to prevent recurrence.

SUPRASPINATUS

Needle size	25 G × ⁵⁄₈ in (0.5 × 16 mm) orange needle or 23 G × 1 in (0.6 × 25 mm) blue needle.

Dose	10 mg triamcinolone acetonide, 0.75 ml local anaesthetic, e.g. 0.25 ml Kenalog®, 0.75 ml 1% lidocaine.

Patient position

Position the patient sitting, supported at an angle of approximately 45°. Medially rotate the shoulder and extend the arm behind the back to expose the superior facet of the greater tuberosity, anteriorly.

Palpation

Supraspinatus inserts into the superior facet of the greater tuberosity. Palpate the anterior border of the acromion and the superior facet on the greater tuberosity. The tendon of supraspinatus runs forward between these two bony points and is approximately as wide as the patient's index finger. Locate the exact site of the lesion by palpation for tenderness along the tendon. Mark a point approximately mid-point of the tender site.

CLINICAL TIP: To locate supraspinatus and infraspinatus (see below), the greater tuberosity provides a useful bony landmark. The greater tuberosity lies in line with the lateral epicondyle at the elbow and this may be used as a point of reference if locating the greater tuberosity proves difficult.

Technique

Insert the needle perpendicular to the teno-osseous junction and deliver the injection by a peppering technique (Figs 5.7 and 5.8).

▶ **FIGURE 5.7**

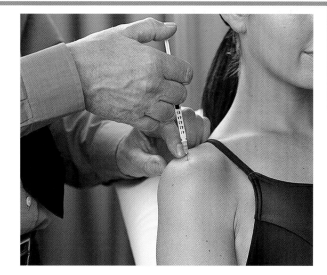

▶ **FIGURE 5.8**

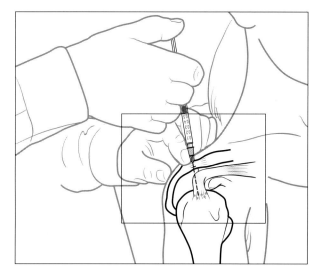

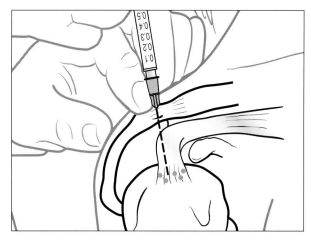

INFRASPINATUS

Needle size	23 G × 1 in (0.6 × 25 mm) or 23 G × 1¼ in (0.6 × 30 mm) blue needle or 21 G × 1½ in (0.8 × 40 mm) green needle, depending on the size of the patient.

Dose	10 mg triamcinolone acetonide, 0.75 ml local anaesthetic, e.g. 0.25 ml Kenalog®, 0.75 ml 1% lidocaine.

Patient position

Place the patient into prone lying, propped up on the elbows, or side lying with the painful side uppermost. In both positions place the shoulder joint into adduction and lateral rotation to expose the middle facet of the greater tuberosity posteriorly.

Palpation

Infraspinatus inserts into the middle facet of the greater tuberosity. Palpate the posterior angle of the acromion and locate the greater tuberosity, below and lateral to this point. The tendon of infraspinatus runs parallel to the spine of the scapula, inserting into the greater tuberosity just below the acromion. It is approximately two fingers wide. Locate the exact site of the lesion by palpating for tenderness along the tendon and mark this point.

Technique

Insert the needle perpendicular to the tendon and deliver the injection by a peppering technique, being sure to cover the whole extent of the lesion (Figs 5.9 and 5.10).

▶ **FIGURE 5.9**

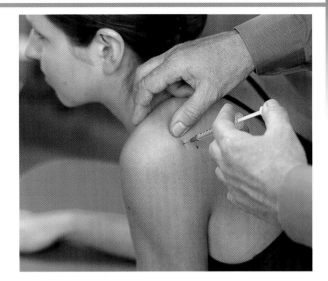

▶ **FIGURE 5.10**

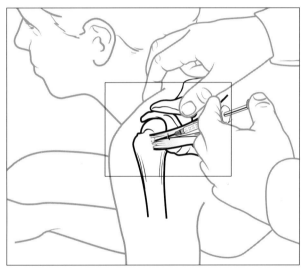

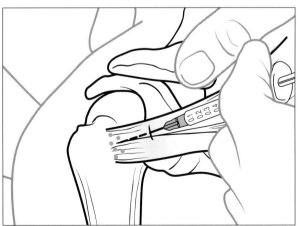

SUBSCAPULARIS

Needle size	23 G × 1 in (0.6 × 25 mm) or 23 G × 1¼ in (0.6 × 30 mm) blue needle.

Dose	10 mg triamcinolone acetonide, 0.75 ml local anaesthetic, e.g. 0.25 ml Kenalog®, 0.75 ml 1% lidocaine.

Patient position

Seat the patient with the arm in the anatomical position and supported on their lap.

Palpation

Subscapularis inserts into the lesser tuberosity and it is approximately three fingers wide, although the thin membranous tendon is not easy to feel. Palpate for the coracoid process and move laterally and slightly down, or identify the bicipital groove and move medially. Both methods will locate the lesser tuberosity. Locate the exact site of the lesion by palpation for tenderness along the tendon. Mark a point approximately mid-point of the tender site.

Technique

Deliver the injection by a peppering technique being sure to cover the full extent of the lesion (Figs 5.11 and 5.12).

A subtendinous bursa lies between the subscapularis tendon and the capsule of the shoulder joint, communicating with the joint. Subscapularis bursitis is difficult to differentiate from tendinitis, but exquisite tenderness on the 'scarf test' and palpation localizes the lesion to the bursa. It can be injected by bolus technique, deep to the tendon.

Patient advice

The patient should be instructed to rest from aggravating activities for a period of up to 2 weeks following the injection.

▶ **FIGURE 5.11**

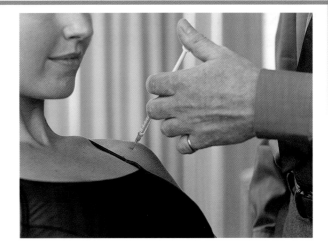

▶ **FIGURE 5.12**

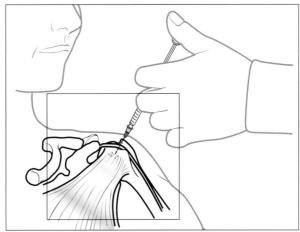

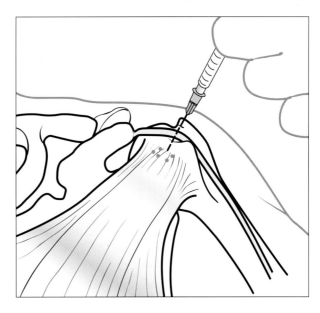

LONG HEAD OF BICEPS IN THE BICIPITAL GROOVE (INTERTUBERCULAR SULCUS)

Indication

Tenosynovitis that may affect the tendon in the bicipital groove. The long head of biceps originates within the capsule of the glenohumeral joint and exits the joint behind the transverse humeral ligament, taking with it an extension of synovial lining into the bicipital groove.

Patient presentation

Pain is felt in the anterior shoulder region usually associated with a history of overuse. On examination, resisted elbow flexion and resisted supination reproduce the pain felt at the shoulder.

Treatment by injection

Tenosynovitis involves inflammation of the double-layered synovial sheath rather than the tendon itself, and adhesions may form between the two layers of the sheath, interfering with function (Cyriax 1982). An accurately placed injection of corticosteroid may be curative.

Needle size	23 G × 1 in (0.6 × 25 mm) or 23 G × 1¼ in (0.6 × 30 mm) blue needle.

Dose	10 mg triamcinolone acetonide, 0.75 ml local anaesthetic, e.g. 0.25 ml Kenalog®, 0.75 ml 1% lidocaine.

Patient position

Position the patient in sitting with the arm supported in the anatomical position.

Palpation

In the anatomical position the bicipital groove faces forward, lying between the greater and lesser tuberosities of the humerus. If in doubt, locate the coracoid process, move down and laterally onto the lesser tuberosity. Lateral to this is the bicipital groove. Mark the area of tenderness, as located by palpation.

Technique

Insert the needle parallel and close to the bicipital groove, approaching from above downwards (Fig. 5.13). The injection is delivered as a bolus into the synovial sheath of the tendon, not into the body of the tendon (Fig. 5.14).

Patient advice

Advise a period of relative rest from aggravating factors for a period of up to 2 weeks.

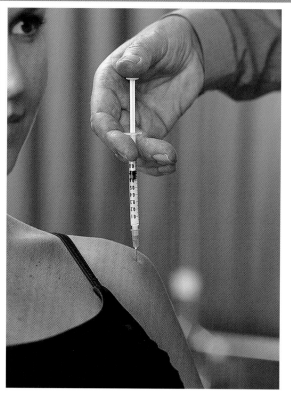

▲ FIGURE 5.13

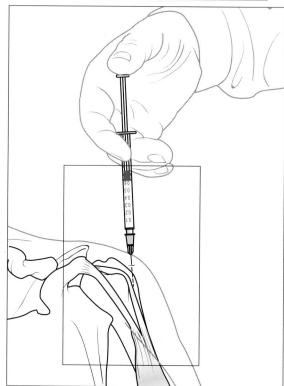

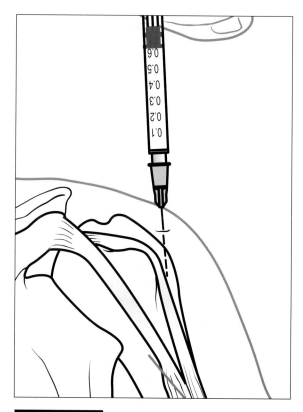

▲ FIGURE 5.14

6 The elbow

ELBOW JOINT

Indication

Arthritis which may be degenerative, traumatic or inflammatory. Inflammatory arthritis, such as rheumatoid, is probably the most common condition to be injected.

Patient presentation

Pain is felt over the elbow and, depending on the severity, may be referred into the forearm. If traumatic in origin the possibility of fracture will need to be excluded.

On examination, there will be a capsular pattern of more limitation of flexion than extension, with the flexion having an abnormal hard end-feel. The superior radio-ulnar joint may be involved, since it shares a common capsule with the elbow joint proper. The capsular pattern at the superior radio-ulnar joint is pain felt at the end of range of both rotations.

Treatment by injection

Despite the complicated anatomical structure of the elbow joint, a bolus injection via the radiohumeral articulation is the easiest intra-articular route. The corticosteroid injection aims to reduce pain and inflammation, allowing recovery of the range of movement.

> **Needle size**
>
> 25 G × ⁵⁄₈ in (0.5 × 16 mm) orange needle for the lateral approach and 23 G × 1 in (0.6 × 25 mm) or 23 G × 1¹⁄₄ in (0.6 × 30 mm) blue needle for the posterior approach.

Dose	20 mg triamcinolone acetonide, 1 ml local anaesthetic, e.g. 2 ml Adcortyl®, 1 ml 1% lidocaine.

Patient position

Seat the patient with the forearm supported in pronation with the elbow at approximately 45° of flexion.

Palpation

Palpate the head of the radius and locate the radiohumeral joint line on the posterolateral aspect. Mark the mid-point of the joint line.

Technique

Insert the needle to lie between the head of the radius and the capitulum of the humerus (Figs 6.1 and 6.2). Deliver the injection as a bolus.

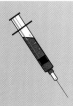

ALTERNATIVE TECHNIQUE: Position the patient with the elbow flexed to 70°. Locate the depression between the olecranon and lateral epicondyle on the posterolateral aspect of the elbow joint. Direct the needle forward and slightly downward and deliver the injection as a bolus.

Patient advice

The patient should be advised to maintain a period of relative rest for approximately 2 weeks following the injection.

▶ **FIGURE 6.1**

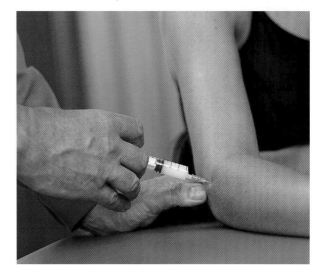

▶ **FIGURE 6.2**

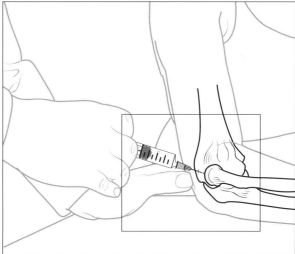

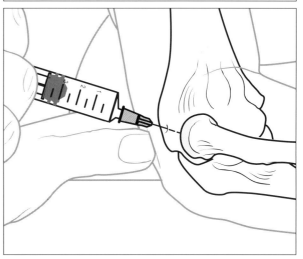

OLECRANON BURSITIS

Indication

Olecranon bursitis (**student's elbow**), is inflammation of the subcutaneous bursa, which is positioned between the upper end of the posterior aspect of the ulna and the skin. Bursitis may be idiopathic, related to trauma, repetitive injury, gout or arthritis, such as rheumatoid (Kumar & Clark 1994). Superficial bursitis such as this may have an infective origin, since it is vulnerable to unrecognized perforating injuries. Diagnosis of this is important before proceeding with the injection.

Patient presentation

Pain is felt over the posterior aspect of the elbow and swelling is both visible and palpable.

On examination there are usually no clinical findings except for the obvious swelling over the olecranon.

Treatment by injection

Injection can be curative, but aspiration to check for the presence of infection is important before proceeding. Clear aspirate is normal; cloudy aspirate indicates possible infection, but bacteriological confirmation may be required.

Needle size	21 G × 1½ in (0.8 × 40 mm) green needle.

Dose	10 mg triamcinolone acetonide, 1 ml local anaesthetic, e.g. 1 ml Adcortyl®, 1 ml 1% lidocaine.

Patient position

Seat the patient with the elbow supported in a degree of flexion.

Palpation

Palpate the obvious swollen bursa and mark a convenient point for inserting the needle.

Technique

Insert the needle into the bursa (Figs 6.3 and 6.4). Aspirate first to check for the presence of infection and if clear, the injection can be delivered as a bolus.

Patient advice

The patient should be advised to avoid further trauma to the bursa.

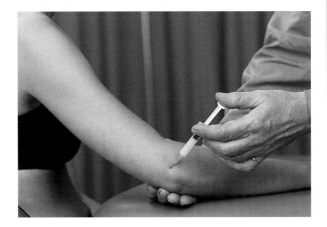

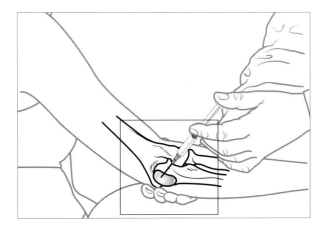

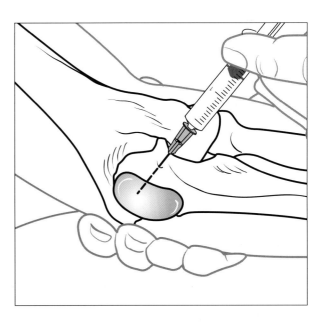

TENNIS ELBOW (LATERAL EPICONDYLITIS)

Indication

Tennis elbow or tendinitis of the wrist extensor muscles at their origin (the enthesis) from the anterior aspect of the lateral epicondyle. The tendon most commonly involved is extensor carpi radialis brevis. Repeated gripping actions may produce traction of fibres at the common extensor origin, leading to microtrauma and inflammation (Foley 1993). Micro- and macroscopic tears lead to the development of fibrous scar tissue and contracture, eventually resulting in degenerative foci and calcification (Coonrad & Hooper 1973, Ernst 1992, Gellman 1992, Noteboom et al 1994). Initial changes in the tendon would seem to be inflammatory and therefore true tendinitis. In chronic long-term lesions the degenerative changes of tendinosis may be more pronounced, making the condition more difficult to deal with. Early treatment, whatever the choice, may prevent the development of chronic lesions and ease pain (Hay et al 1999).

Patient presentation

The patient complains of a gradual increase in pain on the lateral aspect of the elbow, which may radiate into the forearm and sometimes into the dorsum of the wrist and hand. Repeated gripping actions aggravate the symptoms and a twinge of pain is often experienced, when the grip will feel weak.

On examination, resisted wrist extension with the elbow extended provokes the symptoms. The exact site of the lesion is located by palpation.

Treatment by injection

There are several possible sites for the lesion, which will be determined by palpation. Involvement of the origin of the common extensor tendon, mainly extensor carpi radialis brevis at the anterior facet of the lateral epicondyle, is the most common, and is the site that may best respond to injection. However, alternative treatment techniques will be discussed below.

Corticosteroid injection aims to reduce the inflammation and pain. Once pain is reduced, normal movement will encourage alignment of fibres and reduce scarring. Given that the condition can progress to being mainly degenerative, treatment, particularly by corticosteroid injection, would seem to be most efficacious in the early inflammatory phase where good results have been shown in the short term (Price et al 1991, Haker & Lundeberg 1993, Sölveborn et al 1995, Assendelft et al 1996, Verhaar et al 1996, Hay et al 1999).

Price et al (1991) reported a more rapid relief of pain and a reduced need for repeated injections with 10 mg triamcinolone over 25 mg hydrocortisone or lidocaine alone in the short term. Injection of 20 mg triamcinolone produced similar results to 10 mg with the higher dosage more likely to produce skin atrophy. The results of their study were not statistically significant.

Needle size	25 G × $^5/_8$ in (0.5 × 16 mm) orange needle.

Dose	10 mg triamcinolone acetonide, 0.75 ml local anaesthetic, e.g. 0.25 ml Kenalog®, 0.75 ml 1% lidocaine.

Patient position

Seat the patient with the forearm supported in full supination, the elbow flexed to approximately 90°. This positions the tendon to run directly forwards from the anterior facet of the lateral epicondyle.

Palpation

Palpate the lateral epicondyle of the humerus. Roll onto the anterior surface and palpate the insertion of the tendon, which should be tender compared with the other side. Mark a point at the mid-point of the tender site.

Technique

Insert the needle from an anterior direction, perpendicular to the facet, and deliver the injection by a peppering technique (Figs 6.5 and 6.6). Ensure that the injection is delivered to the target tissue and not superficially, which could lead to the complication of local soft tissue atrophy and/or pigmentary changes.

The teno-osseous junction is just one possible site of the lesion, albeit the most common (Cyriax 1982, Cyriax and Cyriax 1983). The other possible sites are the origin of extensor carpi radialis longus from the lower third of the lateral supracondylar ridge, the body of the tendon lying over the head of the radius and the muscle belly. All traditionally respond to physiotherapeutic measures. Techniques such as deep transverse friction massage and Mill's manipulation, electrotherapy and acupuncture, to name a few, are other possible treatment approaches for the common extensor origin site (Cyriax & Cyriax 1983, Cyriax 1984, Kesson & Atkins 1998).

Patient advice

The patient should be advised to maintain a period of relative rest for approximately 2 weeks following the injection. Addressing the cause of the problem is probably the most important issue. Sporting advice may be appropriate in terms of looking at training regimes and grip size. Workstations may need adjusting and breaks from repetitive activities should be strongly encouraged. Counterforce braces (clasps, bandages or strapping) may be helpful.

▶ **FIGURE 6.5**

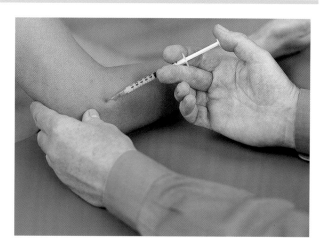

▶ **FIGURE 6.6**

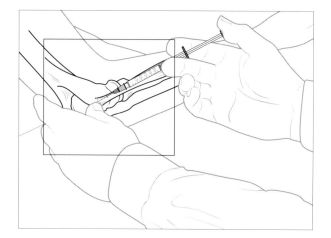

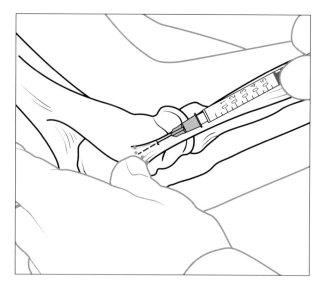

CLINICAL TIP: A branch of the radial nerve, the posterior interosseous nerve, passes between the two heads of the supinator muscle at the elbow. Entrapment of the nerve may be a factor in the resistant tennis elbow. Full assessment to address all causes is essential.

GOLFER'S ELBOW (MEDIAL EPICONDYLITIS)

Indication

Golfer's elbow or tendinitis of the wrist flexor muscles at their origin from the anterior aspect of the medial epicondyle. The aetiology and disease process is similar to that of tennis elbow (*see* p. 70), although Golfer's elbow is not as commonly encountered. The principal site of the lesion is at the teno-osseous junction (the enthesis) of the common flexor tendon but, less commonly, the lesion may be seen a little further distally, in the musculotendinous junction.

Patient presentation

The patient complains of a gradual onset of medial elbow pain, often well localized to the medial epicondyle, although symptoms may be referred more distally. Onset is associated with overuse activities and the symptoms are provoked by use.

On examination, resisted testing of the wrist flexors with the elbow placed in extension is positive, and palpation will locate the exact site of the lesion.

Treatment by injection

Like tennis elbow, early injection can be curative, but the reason for the onset must be determined and the aggravating actions avoided to prevent recurrence. It is the teno-osseous site which responds well to injection (Cyriax & Cyriax 1983).

Needle size	25 G × ⁵/₈ in (0.5 × 16 mm) orange needle or 23 G × 1 in (0.6 × 25 mm) blue needle.

Dose	10 mg triamcinolone acetonide, 0.75 ml local anaesthetic, e.g. 0.25 ml Kenalog®, 0.75 ml 1% lidocaine.

Patient position

Place the patient sitting, with the elbow extended over a pillow and in supination.

Palpation

Palpate the medial epicondyle of the humerus and move round onto its anterior aspect to palpate the origin of the common flexor tendon, identifying the area of maximum tenderness, compared with the other side. Mark a point approximately at the mid-point of the tender site.

Technique

Insert the needle perpendicular to the anterior facet of the medial epicondyle and deliver the injection by a peppering technique (Figs 6.7 and 6.8).

CLINICAL TIP: The ulnar nerve lies posterior to the medial epicondyle of the humerus, but the suggested approach should prevent injection into the nerve itself. Stahl and Kaufman (1997) describe an accidental injury to the ulnar nerve following injection for medial epicondylitis in a patient with undetected recurrent dislocation of the ulnar nerve.

Patient advice

The patient is advised to rest from aggravating factors for up to 2 weeks. As with tennis elbow, it is most important to address the cause of the lesion. The teno-osseous junction (the enthesis) is one site for golfer's elbow, and physio-therapeutic modalities such as deep friction massage and electrotherapy are alternative techniques for treating this lesion. A lesion may exist at the musculo-tendinous junction, but this traditionally responds to physiotherapeutic modalities alone, e.g. transverse friction massage (Cyriax & Cyriax 1983, Cyriax 1984, Kesson & Atkins 1998).

▶ **FIGURE 6.7**

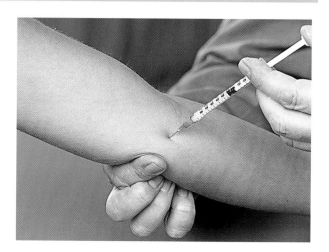

▶ **FIGURE 6.8**

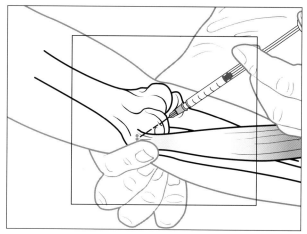

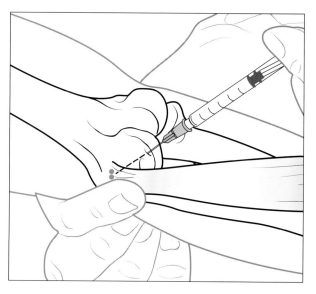

BICEPS TENDON INSERTION AT THE RADIAL TUBEROSITY

Indication

Tendinitis of the insertion of the biceps tendon at the radial tuberosity. This usually arises from overuse and may be difficult to differentially diagnose from inflammation of the subtendinous bursa at this site.

Patient presentation

The patient complains of pain localized to the elbow.

On examination of the elbow joint, resisted elbow flexion and resisted supination reproduce the patient's pain. Involvement of the subtendinous bursa may be indicated by a muddle of signs, e.g. pain on resisted elbow flexion, passive elbow extension and passive pronation, all of which squeeze the inflamed bursa.

Treatment by injection

Since a lesion in either the tendon or the bursa lies deeply, injection of corticosteroid is the treatment of choice.

Needle size	23 G × 1 in (0.6 × 25 mm) blue needle.

Dose	10 mg triamcinolone acetonide, 0.75 ml local anaesthetic, e.g. 0.25 ml Kenalog®, 0.75 ml 1% lidocaine.

Patient position

Position the patient in prone lying, with the arm at the side resting in the anatomical position. Fix the humerus to avoid changing the position of the glenohumeral joint and carefully pronate the extended forearm. This rotates the forearm to bring the radial tuberosity to lie posteriorly.

Palpation

Locate the radial tuberosity, which is lying between the radius and ulna approximately 2 cm distal to the radiohumeral joint line. Mark the principal point of tenderness.

Technique

Insert the needle between the radius and ulna, at the point of maximum tenderness, until the resistance of the tendinous insertion is felt (Figs 6.9 and 6.10). Deliver the injection by a peppering technique to cover both the insertion of the tendon and the subtendinous bursa.

Patient advice

Advise the patient to maintain a period of relative rest for up to 2 weeks after the injection. As with all overuse lesions, eliminating the causative factors will prevent recurrence.

▶ FIGURE 6.9

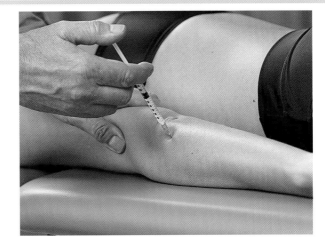

▶ FIGURE 6.10

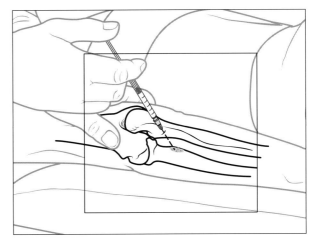

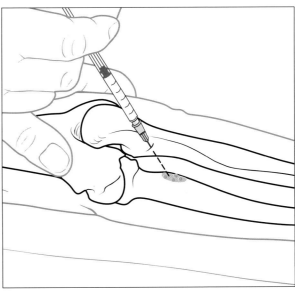

7 The wrist and hand

INFERIOR (DISTAL) RADIO-ULNAR JOINT

Indication

Arthritis, most commonly rheumatoid arthritis at this joint, although degenerative and traumatic arthritis may also cause symptoms.

Patient presentation

The patient complains of pain felt in the lower forearm.

On examination, a capsular pattern is present with pain reproduced at the end of both extremes of passive pronation and supination. Limitation of these movements is not usually found, except in advanced cases of arthritis.

Treatment by injection

A bolus injection of corticosteroid aims to reduce inflammation and pain.

Needle size	23 G × 1 in (0.6 × 25 mm) blue needle.

Dose	10 mg triamcinolone acetonide, 0.75 ml local anaesthetic, e.g. 0.25 ml Kenalog®, 0.75 ml 1% lidocaine.

Patient position

Position the patient sitting, with the forearm supported in pronation.

Palpation

On the dorsal surface, the inferior radio-ulnar joint lies approximately 1.5 cm from the ulnar styloid process. The joint can be glided passively to confirm its position. Mark a point over the mid-point of the joint line.

Technique

Insert the needle via the dorsal surface of the inferior radio-ulnar joint line, angling it if necessary to allow for the curvature of the articular surfaces (Figs 7.1 and 7.2). Deliver the injection as a bolus once the needle is intracapsular.

Patient advice

The patient is advised to maintain a period of relative rest for up to 2 weeks following the injection.

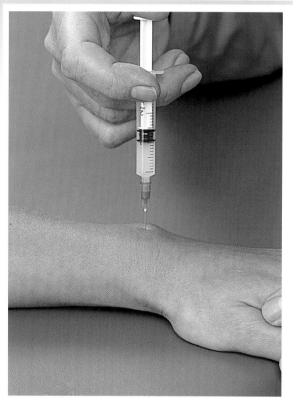

▲ FIGURE 7.1

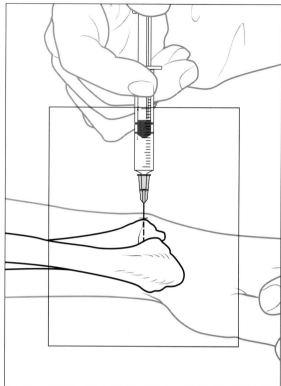

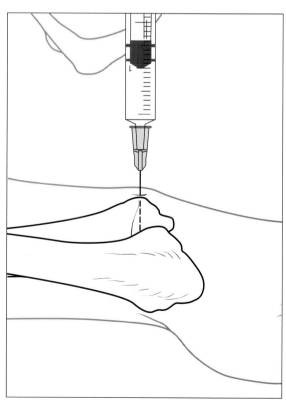

▲ FIGURE 7.2

WRIST JOINT

Indication

Arthritis, most commonly rheumatoid arthritis at this joint, although degenerative and traumatic arthritis may also cause symptoms. If the lesion is due to trauma, fracture of one of the carpal bones, usually the scaphoid, should be excluded.

Patient presentation

The patient presents with pain felt locally at the wrist. There may be a history of trauma, or if due to inflammatory arthritis the patient may have other joint involvement.

On examination the joint may be swollen, and heat and synovial thickening may be palpated at the wrist. Assessment by selective tension will reveal a capsular pattern of equal limitation of flexion and extension.

Treatment by injection

The aim of treatment by corticosteroid injection is to reduce inflammation and pain.

Needle size	23 G × 1 in (0.6 × 25 mm) blue needle.

Dose	20 mg triamcinolone acetonide, 1 ml local anaesthetic, e.g. 2 ml Adcortyl®, 1 ml 1% lidocaine.

Patient position

Position the patient sitting, with the forearm supported in pronation.

Palpation

Palpate the radiocarpal joint line on the dorsal surface of the wrist; select and mark a point on either side of the extensor carpi radialis brevis tendon.

Technique

Insert the needle into the joint angled slightly proximally to allow for the curvature of the articular surfaces (Figs 7.3 and 7.4). The proximal carpal

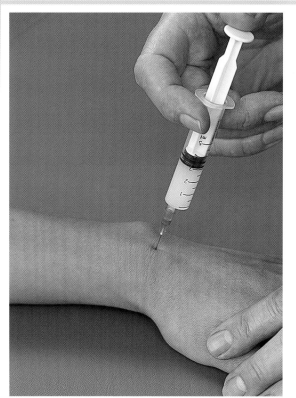

▲ **FIGURE 7.3**

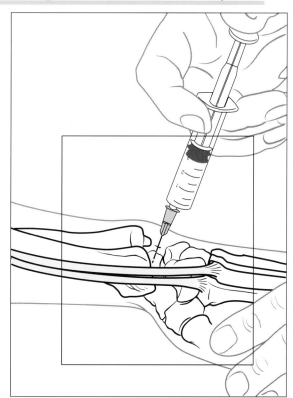

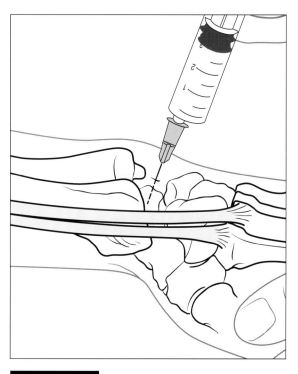

▲ **FIGURE 7.4**

bones are slightly convex and the lower end of the radius is concave. Deliver the injection by a bolus technique once intracapsular.

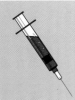

ALTERNATIVE TECHNIQUES:
1. In the wrist affected by rheumatoid arthritis, it may not be possible to introduce the needle into the joint capsule. Palpate for the areas of tenderness around the wrist and use two or three separate needle insertions to pepper the areas of synovial thickening (changing the needle for each insertion). This technique may be painful for the patient.
2. Palpate the radio-ulnar joint line and insert the needle immediately distal to the ulnar styloid process. Deliver the injection by a bolus technique.

Patient advice

The patient is advised to maintain a period of relative rest for up to 2 weeks following the injection. If pain is severe, a supporting splint may be worn.

TRAPEZIO-FIRST METACARPAL JOINT (FIRST CARPOMETACARPAL JOINT)

Indication

Arthritis, which may be inflammatory arthritis, but more commonly it results from an overuse activity that precipitates a traumatic arthritis in an already degenerate joint.

Patient presentation

The patient complains of pain felt locally at the base of the thumb, which is aggravated by activities that involve compression of the joint, e.g. writing and gripping. The condition commonly affects middle-aged women (Livengood 1992).

On examination the capsular pattern of limited extension at the trapezio-first metacarpal joint is present.

Treatment by injection

Injection may be successful for inflammatory, degenerative or traumatic arthritis of this joint. In the symptomatic degenerate joint, physiotherapeutic modalities such as mobilization and transverse friction massage to the capsular ligaments can give good symptomatic relief (Cyriax & Cyriax 1983, Cyriax 1984, Kesson and Atkins 1998).

Needle size	25 G × ⅝ in (0.5 × 16 mm) orange needle.

Dose	10 mg triamcinolone acetonide, 0.25 ml local anaesthetic, e.g. 0.25 ml Kenalog®, 0.25 ml 1% lidocaine.

Patient position

Position the patient sitting, with the forearm supported.

Palpation

Identify the first metacarpal. Run your thumb down this bone to its proximal end in the anatomical snuffbox and locate the joint line. The patient may be able to help identification and facilitate the injection by applying a little distraction to the joint. Mark the mid-point of the joint line.

Technique

Insert the needle perpendicularly into the joint and deliver the injection as a bolus once the needle is intracapsular (Figs 7.5 and 7.6).

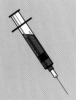

ALTERNATIVE TECHNIQUE: Position the thumb in extension and adduction. Identify the joint line anteriorly on the palmar surface, through the thenar eminence. Insert the needle into the joint and deliver the injection by a bolus. This approach may be useful if the patient has had long-standing symptoms and some wasting of the thenar muscles.

CLINICAL TIP: Osteophytes around the degenerate joint may impede the injection via either of the approaches given. The gentle distraction of the joint facilitates the needle insertion into the joint space.

Patient advice

Advise the patient to maintain a period of relative rest from the aggravating factors for up to 2 weeks.

▶ FIGURE 7.5

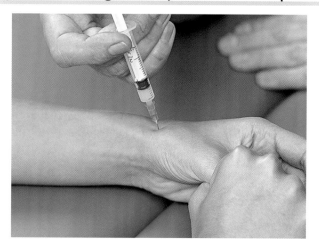

▶ FIGURE 7.6

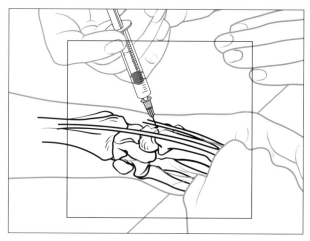

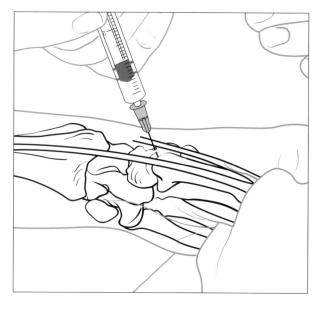

METACARPOPHALANGEAL JOINTS AND INTERPHALANGEAL JOINTS

Indication

Arthritis, which may be degenerative, inflammatory or traumatic.

Patient presentation

The patient will be able to localize their pain to the particular joint(s) involved.
On examination, the capsular pattern of limitation of movement will confirm the diagnosis. For the metacarpophalangeal joints the capsular pattern is limitation of radial deviation and extension, while the interphalangeal joints demonstrate an equal limitation of flexion and extension.

Treatment by injection

Corticosteroid injection aims to reduce the inflammation and give effective pain relief.

Needle size	25 G × ⅝ in (0.5 × 16 mm) orange needle.

Dose	5–10 mg triamcinolone acetonide, 0.25 ml local anaesthetic, e.g. 0.25 ml Kenalog®, 0.25 ml 1% lidocaine.

Patient position

Position the patient sitting, with the hand supported comfortably.

Palpation

Locate the symptomatic joint by palpation and identify the joint line. Mark a point on the dorsolateral aspect of the joint line.

Technique

Insert the needle into the relevant joint via a dorsolateral approach, avoiding the dorsal digital expansion (Figs 7.7, 7.8, 7.9 and 7.10). Once intracapsular, the injection can be delivered as a bolus.

Patient advice

Advise the patient to maintain a period of relative rest for up to 2 weeks after the injection.

▶ **FIGURE 7.7**

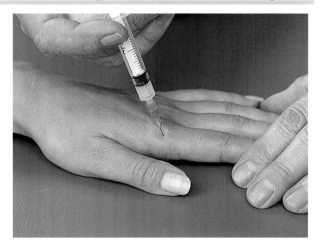

▶ **FIGURE 7.8**

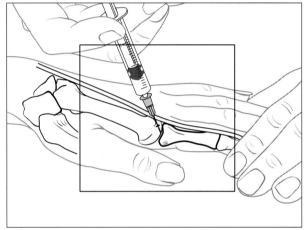

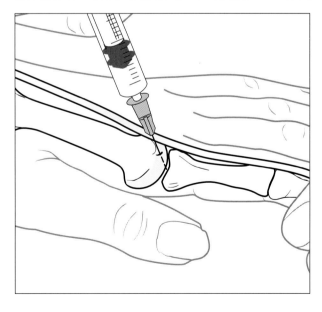

▶ **FIGURE 7.9**

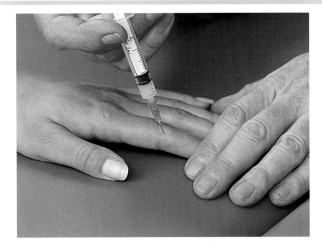

▶ **FIGURE 7.10**

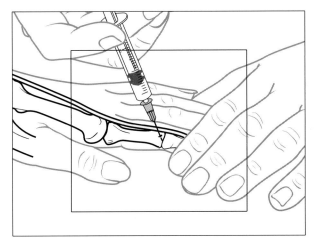

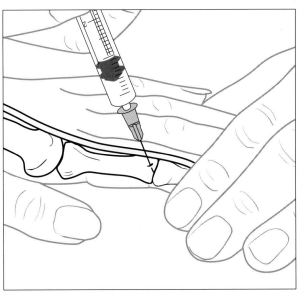

RADIAL AND ULNAR COLLATERAL LIGAMENTS

Indication

Ligamentous sprain due to a single traumatic incident or repetitive micro-trauma through overuse.

Patient presentation

The patient complains of pain well localized to the lateral or medial aspects of the wrist joint, respectively.

On examination, a non-capsular pattern of pain on passive ulnar deviation will be positive in a sprain of the radial collateral ligament, while passive radial deviation will be positive in a sprain of the ulnar collateral ligament.

Treatment by injection

A corticosteroid injection may be curative or, alternatively, physiotherapeutic methods including mobilization by transverse friction massage may be used.

Needle size	25 G × ⁵/₈ in (0.5 × 16 mm) orange needle.

Dose	10 mg triamcinolone acetonide, 0.25 ml local anaesthetic, e.g. 0.25 ml Kenalog®, 0.25 ml 1% lidocaine.

Patient position

Position the patient comfortably in sitting, with the hand supported.

Palpation

Palpate for the area of tenderness over the ligament and mark this point.

Technique

Insert the needle perpendicular to the ligament (Figs 7.11, 7.12, 7.13 and 7.14) and deliver the injection to the affected area by peppering technique.

Patient advice

Advise the patient to maintain a period of relative rest for up to 2 weeks after the injection.

▶ **FIGURE 7.11**

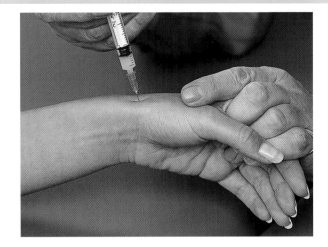

▶ **FIGURE 7.12**

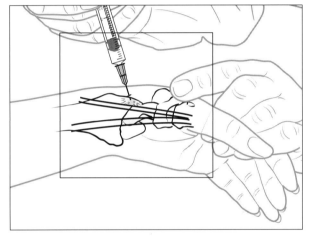

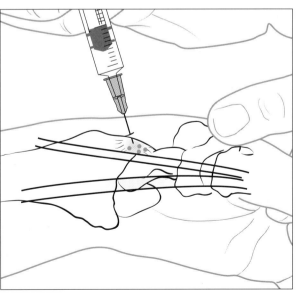

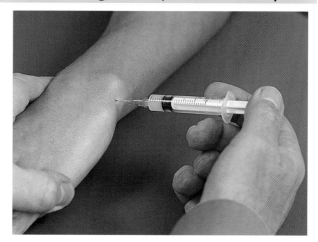

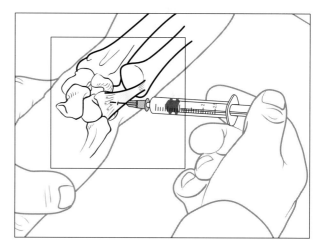

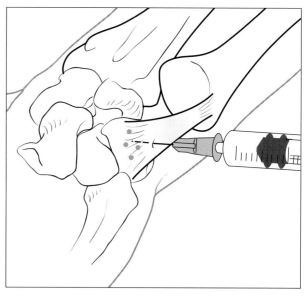

CARPAL TUNNEL

Indication

Compression of the median nerve in the carpal tunnel. The median nerve passes through a fibro-osseous tunnel formed by the overlying flexor retinaculum and the underlying carpal bones. This is a restricted space, being occupied by the superficial and deep flexor tendons to the digits, as well as the median nerve and vessels. Any reduction in the space causes compression of the median nerve and produces symptoms (see below). Intrinsic factors such as inflammation and swelling, or extrinsic factors such as trauma or repetitive occupational and leisure activities, may be the reason for the condition. It is more common in women between the ages of 40 and 60 years (Norris 1993, Kumar & Clark 1994) and the syndrome may also be associated with diabetes, myxoedema, pregnancy and rheumatoid arthritis. In advanced cases, the muscles of the thenar eminence may become weak, particularly abductor pollicis brevis, which causes the first metacarpal to fall back into the same plane as the other metacarpals.

Patient presentation

The history generally substantiates the diagnosis. The patient complains of aching and burning pain, with tingling or numbness of the fingertips. Paraesthesia is reported on the palmar aspect of the radial three and a half digits. Smith and Wernick (1994) reported 70% of patients feeling numbness at night and 40% complaining of pain radiating proximally into the lower forearm, with paraesthesia felt simultaneously in the fingers. The patient may be woken at night by the symptoms and gain relief by shaking or rubbing the hands (Cailliet 1990).

On examination, wasting of the thenar eminence may be observed and weakness experienced in advanced cases. Traditionally Tinel's test (tapping over the flexor retinaculum) and Phalen's test (the application of sustained compression to the median nerve by maintaining the wrist in a position of flexion) are used to elicit the reported paraesthesia and to diagnose carpal tunnel syndrome (Hoppenfeld 1976, Otto & Wehbé 1986, Cailliet 1990, Vargas Busquets 1994). However, false-positive and false-negative results are not uncommon.

Treatment by injection

Injection of corticosteroid into the carpal tunnel may reduce the inflammation and swelling associated with the compressed nerve and reduce or eliminate the symptoms for the patient. The more advanced cases, with muscle weakness and wasting, should be referred for surgical opinion.

Needle size	23 G × 1 in (0.6 × 25 mm) or 23 G × 1¼ in (0.6 × 30 mm) blue needle.

Dose	20 mg triamcinolone acetonide, e.g. 0.5 ml Kenalog®.
	The injection is not particularly painful for the patient and a small volume of concentrated corticosteroid is advised. The addition of local anaesthetic serves no purpose here and its addition would increase the volume of the injection unnecessarily.

Patient position

Position the patient sitting, with the wrist supported in extension and the forearm supinated.

Palpation

Observe the three skin creases, which are generally visible on the palmar aspect of the lower forearm. Note the position of palmaris longus, which gives an approximate position of the underlying median nerve.

CLINICAL TIP: If palmaris longus is absent, ask the patient to oppose the thumb and little finger. The mid-line crease produced between the thenar and hypothenar eminences gives the approximate position of the median nerve in the carpal tunnel.

Mark a point between the middle and distal wrist creases, to the ulnar side of palmaris longus (or the middle crease as identified above).

Technique

Insert the needle between the middle and distal wrist creases, to the ulnar side of the palmaris longus tendon, which ensures that you do not make contact with the median nerve (Fig. 7.15). Angle the needle approximately parallel with the direction of the flexor tendons in the carpal tunnel. Advance the needle between the flexor tendons until you judge it to rest beyond the distal wrist crease and therefore within the carpal tunnel (Fig. 7.16). Deliver the injection as a bolus.

CLINICAL TIP: If you grip the syringe gently, the needle will glide into the carpal tunnel parallel to the tendons. As you position the needle for injection, check with the patient that they are not experiencing paraesthesia, to avoid injecting into the nerve itself.

▶ FIGURE 7.15

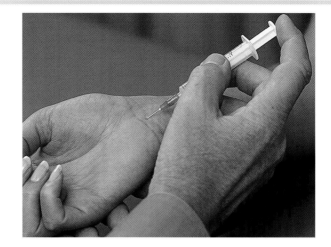

▶ FIGURE 7.16

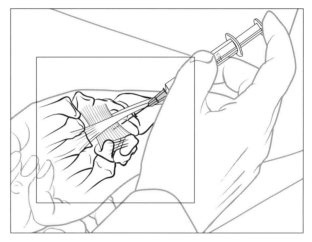

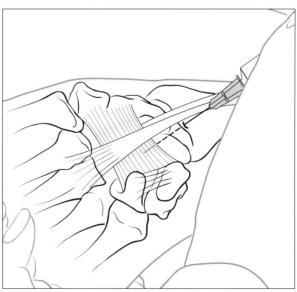

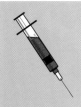

ALTERNATIVE TECHNIQUES:

1. Position the patient with the forearm supinated and insert the needle $^1/_2$ inch distal to the distal wrist crease, aiming down and towards the wrist joint. Once under the flexor retinaculum, inject as a bolus.
2. Position the patient with the wrist in a degree of extension and the forearm supinated. Insert the needle just proximal to the distal wrist crease immediately to the radial side of palmaris longus (if palmaris longus is absent, see above). Advance the needle between the flexor tendons until you judge it to rest within the carpal tunnel. Deliver the injection as a bolus.

Patient advice

It is most important to ascertain the cause of this lesion and to eliminate these factors to prevent recurrence. The patient should maintain a period of relative rest for up to 2 weeks following the injection and avoid all aggravating factors. A wrist-supporting splint may be helpful.

Carpal tunnel syndrome may be part of a wider scenario and it may be necessary to eliminate causes in the cervical spine and those involving adverse neural tension (pathoneurodynamics).

CLINICAL TIP: The use of corticosteroid injection for carpal tunnel syndrome in pregnancy is not recommended.

TRIGGER FINGER OR TRIGGER THUMB

Indication

A 'catching' or 'triggering' phenomenon of a flexor tendon in its sheath. The superficial and deep flexor tendons pass through osseo-aponeurotic canals, which are formed by the phalanges, their joints and the digital fibrous sheaths. Midway between the proximal and intermediate phalanges is a stronger thickening of transverse fibres known as an annular pulley (Williams et al 1989). These pulleys prevent bowstringing of the tendons and enhance tendon efficiency. The flexor tendons receive maximum stress at the pulley level with the metacarpophalangeal joint, and nodules form in long-standing conditions (Otto & Wehbé 1986, Lloyd Davies 1998).

Patient presentation

The patient complains of a localized, painful, 'snapping' sensation as a flexor tendon catches in a thickened area of its sheath on flexion, and is suddenly released during forced extension (Smith & Wernick 1994, Murphy et al 1995).

There may be little to find on examination, but an area of thickening may be observed or there may be a palpable nodule.

Treatment by injection

Injection of corticosteroid may be curative and aims to restore painless, smooth movement at the finger (Anderson & Kaye 1991, Lambert et al 1992, Murphy et al 1995, Speed 2001).

Needle size	25 G × ⁵⁄₈ in (0.5 × 16 mm) orange needle.

Dose	10 mg triamcinolone acetonide, 0.25 ml local anaesthetic, e.g. 0.25 ml Kenalog®, 0.25 ml 1% lidocaine.

Patient position

Position the patient in sitting, with the hand supported.

Palpation

Palpate the symptomatic digit for the area of pain and thickening. Mark the mid-point.

Technique

Insert the needle into the thickened nodule of the affected tendon on the palmar surface (Figs 7.17 and 7.18). Angle the needle approximately 45°, distally or proximally, with the bevel of the needle parallel to the tendon. Avoid injecting into the tendon itself by withdrawing back from the tendon slightly until a loss of resistance is appreciated, and deliver the injection by peppering technique.

Patient advice

Advise the patient to maintain a period of relative rest for up to 2 weeks after the injection.

▶ **FIGURE 7.17**

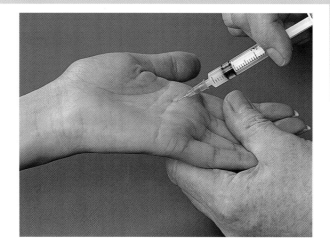

▶ **FIGURE 7.18**

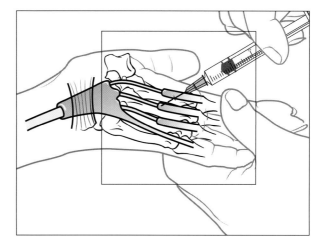

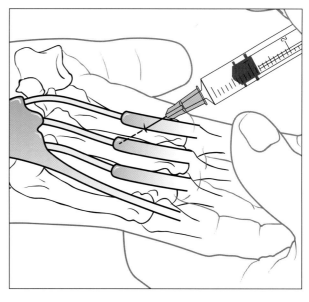

DE QUERVAIN'S TENOSYNOVITIS

Indication

Tenosynovitis due to inflammation of the shared synovial sheath of abductor pollicis longus and extensor pollicis brevis in the first extensor compartment at the wrist. The condition may be complicated by thickening and scarring of the sheath, and occasionally a ganglion may be associated with the chronic condition (Tan et al 1994, Klug 1995).

Patient presentation

The onset can be due to trauma, but overuse more commonly causes a gradual onset of pain felt on the radial side of the wrist. The area over the radial styloid may feel tender to palpation. An audible crepitus may be present on movements of the thumb.

On examination, a localized, thickened area over the tendons may be observed. Symptoms will be reproduced on testing resisted abduction and extension of the thumb. Passive movements may also be painful as the tendons move through the thickened, inflamed sheath. Finkelstein's test (flexion of the thumb across the palm with ulnar deviation at the wrist increasing the angulation of the tendon) produces the pain and is said to be pathognomonic of de Quervain's tenosynovitis (Otto and Wehbé 1986, Shea et al 1991, Livengood 1992, Elliott 1992, Rettig 1994).

Treatment by injection

An injection of corticosteroid aims to reduce inflammation, swelling and pain. If the condition is resistant to treatment by injection, physiotherapeutic modalities may be considered or the patient may need a surgical opinion.

Needle size	25 G × ⁵⁄₈ in (0.5 × 16 mm) orange needle.

Dose	10 mg triamcinolone acetonide, 0.75 ml local anaesthetic, e.g. 0.25 ml Kenalog®, 0.75 ml 1% lidocaine.

Patient position

Position the patient in sitting, with the wrist supported. Hold the thumb in a degree of flexion and the wrist in ulnar deviation and slight extension.

Palpation

Locate the triangular 'gap' between abductor pollicis longus and extensor pollicis brevis tendons at the base of the first metacarpal. Mark this point.

Technique

Insert the needle between and parallel to the two tendons, delivering the injection as a bolus, into the common sheath (Figs 7.19 and 7.20).

Patient advice

Advise the patient to maintain a period of relative rest for up to two weeks after the injection. As the lesion is due to overuse activities, the causative factors should be addressed to prevent recurrence.

FIGURE 7.19

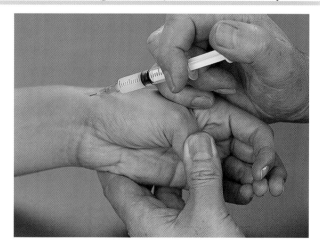

FIGURE 7.20

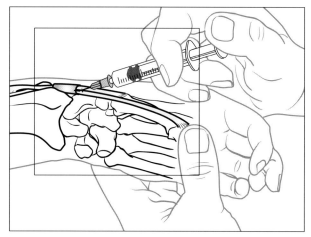

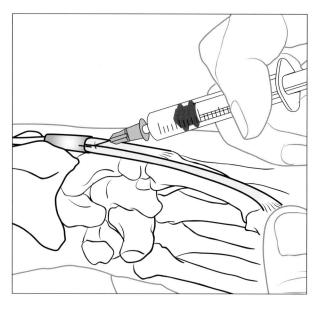

WRIST EXTENSOR AND FLEXOR TENDON LESIONS

Indication

Tenosynovitis or tendinitis. Tenosynovitis may affect the tendons as they cross the wrist and hand protected by their synovial sheaths. Tendinitis may be present at the teno-osseous junction, i.e. the point of insertion of the tendon into the bone.

Patient presentation

These are most frequently overuse lesions, with the patient complaining of a gradual onset of pain which is well localized.

On examination, a resisted test, appropriate for the individual tendon, will be positive. In the case of tenosynovitis, the opposite passive movement may also be painful as the tendon is pushed or pulled through its inflamed sheath.

Treatment by injection

Injection of corticosteroid solution aims to reduce inflammation and relieve pain.

Needle size	25 G × $^5/_8$ in (0.5 × 16 mm) orange needle.

Dose	10 mg triamcinolone acetonide, 0.75 ml local anaesthetic, e.g. 0.25 ml Kenalog®, 0.75 ml 1% lidocaine.

Patient position

Position the patient sitting, with the hand supported.

Palpation

Locate the area of tenderness and mark the central point.

Technique

At the teno-osseous junction deliver the injection by a peppering technique. For tenosynovitis the injection is delivered as a bolus between the tendon and its sheath.

EXTENSOR CARPI RADIALIS LONGUS AND BREVIS

Pain is reproduced on resisted wrist extension and resisted radial deviation. Extensor carpi radialis longus inserts into the radial side of the base of the second metacarpal and extensor carpi radialis brevis into the radial side of the base of the third metacarpal. At the teno-osseous site the injection can be delivered by a peppering technique (Figs 7.21 and 7.22). A lesion involving the common sheath of these tendons is not common, but if present, injection is delivered between the tendon and its sheath by a bolus technique.

▶ **FIGURE 7.21**

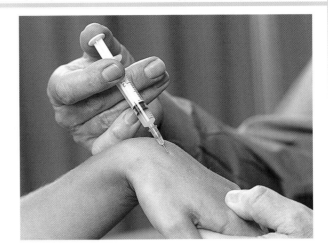

▶ **FIGURE 7.22**

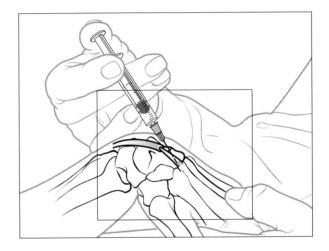

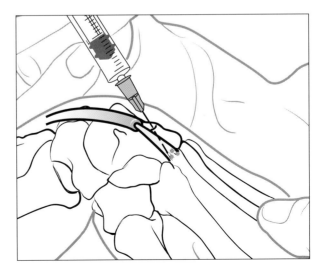

EXTENSOR CARPI ULNARIS

Pain is reproduced on resisted wrist extension and resisted ulnar deviation. The tendon inserts into the base of the fifth metacarpal, where an injection may be delivered using a peppering technique. If the lesion is tenosynovitis, either as the tendon crosses the wrist or in the groove between the head of the ulna and the ulnar styloid process, the injection is delivered between the tendon and its sheath using a bolus technique (Figs 7.23 and 7.24).

▶ **FIGURE 7.23**

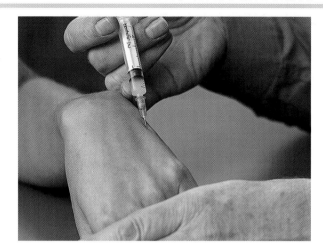

▶ **FIGURE 7.24**

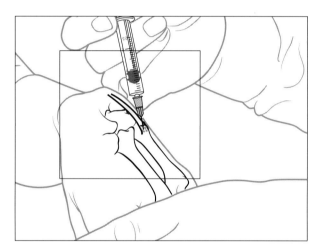

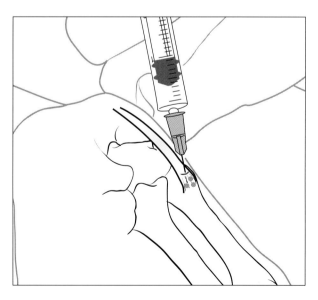

FLEXOR CARPI ULNARIS

Pain is reproduced on resisted wrist flexion and resisted ulnar deviation. The tendon may be affected at its teno-osseous junction either proximal or distal to the pisiform. Injection is delivered by a peppering technique to the area found to be tender to palpation (Figs 7.25 and 7.26).

CLINICAL TIP: The ulnar artery and nerve pass into the hand lateral to the pisiform bone.

▶ FIGURE 7.25

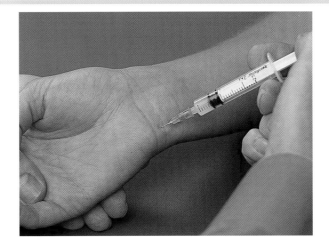

▶ FIGURE 7.26

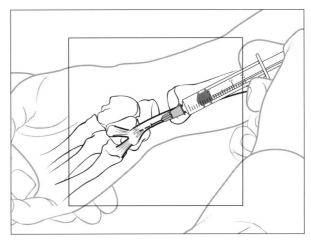

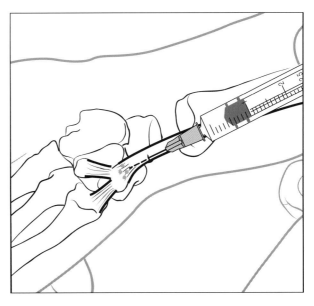

8 The hip

HIP JOINT

Indication

Arthritis, most commonly acute episodes of degenerative arthritis, but may also be indicated in inflammatory arthritis or possibly traumatic arthritis. Primary degenerative osteoarthrosis is common and is said to occur in 50% of the population over the age of 60 years (Kumar & Clark 1994). Men and women are equally affected (Dieppe 1995).

Patient presentation

The patient complains of a gradual onset of pain and loss of mobility. The pain may be felt in the area of the L3 dermatome, i.e. the upper buttock, groin, or referred into the medial aspect and front of the thigh and leg as far as the medial malleolus. The more distally the pain is felt, the more irritable the lesion. Pain may be associated with activity and/or rest. X-ray changes are not a good indicator of the symptoms, as joint changes may be seen long before symptoms present and vice versa.

On examination, a capsular pattern of limited movement exists, limited medial rotation, flexion, abduction and extension. The limited movements will have lost their normal elastic end-feel and will feel hard at the end of range.

Treatment by injection

Osteoarthrosis progresses with periods of exacerbation and remission (Dieppe 1995). A corticosteroid injection may give symptomatic relief and improve function for the patient. It may postpone the need for surgical intervention. As mentioned above, inflammatory arthritis such as rheumatoid arthritis may also benefit from an intra-articular injection.

Needle size	20 G × 3¹/₂ in (0.9 × 90 mm) spinal needle.

Dose	40 mg triamcinolone acetonide, 1 ml local anaesthetic, e.g. 4 ml Adcortyl®, 1 ml 1% lidocaine.
	Some authorities recommend the use of much larger volumes of local anaesthetic, to cause distension of the hip joint capsule.

Patient position

Position the patient in side lying, with the painful leg uppermost, supported in neutral by a pillow.

Palpation

Palpate the greater trochanter (the large quadrangular, bony prominence on the lateral aspect of the upper femur), approximately one hand's breadth below the iliac crest. Grasp the greater trochanter with thumb, index and middle fingers, lift the leg passively into abduction to relax the iliotibial tract and feel the dip above the top of the greater trochanter with your index finger. Mark a point just proximal to your index finger and replace the leg into the neutral position.

Technique

Insert the needle at the point marked and aim vertically down toward the neck of the femur, until contact is made with bone (Figs 8.1 and 8.2). Since the fibrous capsule of the hip joint surrounds the neck of the femur, the needle will be intracapsular once this contact is made. Deliver the injection as a bolus.

 CLINICAL TIP: Since septic arthritis of the hip is a very serious complication, a 'no-touch' technique is absolutely essential to prevent infection. Some authorities advocate injecting the hip joint under surgical conditions.

 CLINICAL TIP: There is some controversy concerning repeated steroid injections into weight-bearing joints and the associated risk of developing steroid arthropathy (Parikh et al 1993, Cameron 1995a). To minimize risk of steroid arthropathy, it is recommended that weight-bearing joints should not be injected more frequently than every 4–6 months.

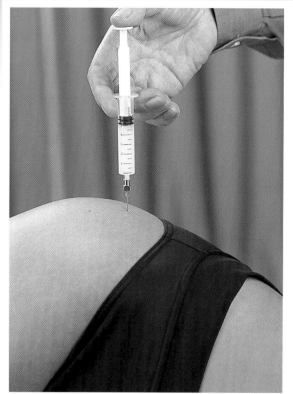

▲ FIGURE 8.1

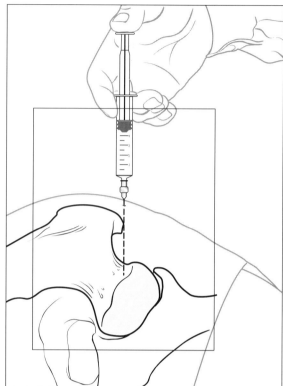

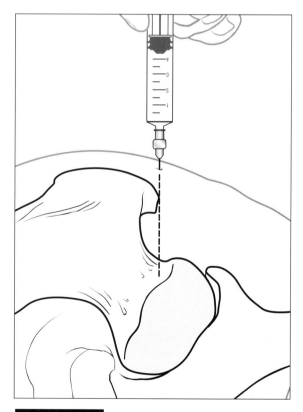

▲ FIGURE 8.2

Patient advice

Advise the patient to maintain a period of relative rest for up to 2 weeks after the injection. Since Chakravarty and Pharoah (1994) showed that 24 hours of complete bed-rest following injection of the knee joint for rheumatoid arthritis produced more prolonged benefit, it may also be appropriate to apply this regime to the hip joint.

PSOAS BURSA (ILIOPSOAS BURSA)

Indication

Psoas bursitis that may be due to repetitive minor trauma or a single traumatic incident, but the bursa's communication with the hip joint means that the condition may be associated with hip joint pathology such as rheumatoid arthritis (Armstrong & Saxton 1972, Meaney et al 1992).

Patient presentation

The patient may complain of a gradual onset of pain, felt in the groin or referred into the L3 dermatome (the upper buttock, the medial aspect and front of the thigh and leg as far as the medial malleolus).

On examination, a non-capsular pattern exists with a 'muddle' of signs characteristic of bursitis, i.e. possibly pain on passive lateral rotation, passive extension and resisted flexion of the hip. Diagnosis is confirmed by combined passive flexion and adduction of the hip, which compresses the bursa against the front of the hip joint.

Treatment by injection

The treatment of choice for psoas bursitis is an injection of a large volume of low-dose local anaesthetic, together with an appropriate amount of corticosteroid. The injection aims to reduce inflammation and to relieve pain.

Needle size	20 G × 3$\frac{1}{2}$ in (0.9 × 90 mm) spinal needle.

Dose	20 mg triamcinolone acetonide, 8 ml local anaesthetic, e.g. 2 ml Adcortyl®, 8 ml 0.5% lidocaine.

Patient position

Position the patient in supine lying, with the groin area exposed.

Palpation

The psoas bursa is a large bursa, measuring approximately 5–7 cm in length and 2–4 cm in width in its normal collapsed state (Underwood et al 1988, Toohey et al 1990, Flanagan et al 1995). It lies between the musculotendinous junction of the iliopsoas muscle and the front of the capsule of the hip joint, protecting the tendon as it winds around the front of the hip joint, to its insertion into the lesser trochanter.

Establishing the position of the bursa for injection is complicated, since it is also associated anteriorly with the neurovascular bundle in the femoral triangle, which must be avoided. Locate and mark the femoral pulse, just distal to the mid-point of the inguinal ligament. The psoas bursa lies deep to the artery. To avoid the neurovascular bundle, move laterally 5 cm and distally 5 cm and mark this point (Fig. 8.3a).

Technique

Insert the needle at the marked point and angle it deeply, medially and proximally towards the bursa, to be deep to the neurovascular bundle (the initial point of palpation recommended above, located by the femoral pulse) (Figs 8.3b and 8.4). On making contact with bone, the needle is now at the front of the hip joint and should be withdrawn slightly so that it is positioned within the psoas bursa. If there is no resistance to the injection, deliver the injection using a bolus technique.

Resistance to the injection may indicate that the bursa is multiloculated with well-defined walls, and it may also contain debris. In this case, deliver the injection by peppering technique, covering the area of the lesion determined by tenderness to palpation (Meaney et al 1992, Cyriax & Cyriax 1983, Kesson & Atkins 1998).

Kerry et al (2000) describe a collaborative approach to diagnosis and treatment of iliopsoas bursitis with corticosteroid injection, ultrasonography and physiotherapy.

Patient advice

Advise the patient to maintain a period of relative rest for up to 2 weeks following the injection. The causative factors should be ascertained and avoided to prevent recurrence.

▶ **FIGURE 8.3a**

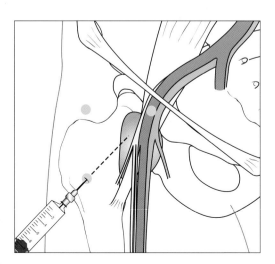

▶ **FIGURE 8.3b**

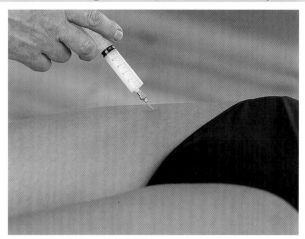

▶ **FIGURE 8.4**

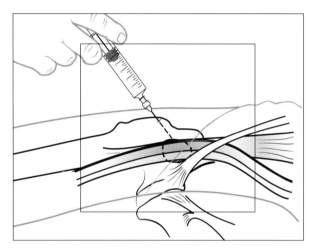

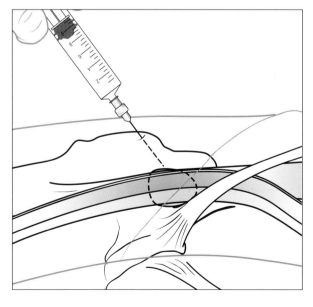

TROCHANTERIC BURSA

Indication

Trochanteric bursitis, usually due to repetitive overuse, although the condition may be associated with tight lateral structures at the hip, such as the iliotibial band, or with lumbar, sacro-iliac or hip joint pathology (Shbeeb et al 1996).

Patient presentation

The patient presents with a gradual onset of pain felt in the lateral thigh.

On examination there are usually no clinical findings, apart from tenderness to palpation over the greater trochanter. Resisted hip abduction and/or passive lateral rotation may provoke the symptoms (Rasmussen and Fano 1985, Shbeeb et al 1996). There may be some muscle tightness on testing for range of joint movement or leg-length inequality as a precipitating factor.

Treatment by injection

Providing the causative factors are also addressed, injection of corticosteroid may be curative and is therefore the treatment of choice (Schapira et al 1986). Shbeeb et al (1996) conducted an observational study of 75 patients with trochanteric bursitis with an injection of either 6, 12 or 24 mg betamethasone. Their results indicated that most patients improved with a single injection, those that received the highest dose of corticosteroid reported longer-term improvement.

Needle size	21 G × 1$^1/_2$ in (0.8 × 40 mm) or 21 G × 2 in (0.8 × 50 mm) green needle.

Dose	20 mg triamcinolone acetonide, 1–3 ml local anaesthetic, e.g. 2 ml Adcortyl®, 1–3 ml 1% lidocaine.

Patient position

Position the patient in supported side lying.

Palpation

The trochanteric bursa caps the greater trochanter, separating the overlying gluteus maximus muscle from the bone as it passes to its insertion into the iliotibial tract and upper femur. The position is similar to the way in which the subacromial bursa caps the greater tuberosity of the humerus. Locate the large, quadrangular greater trochanter and palpate for an area of tenderness over its superolateral aspect. Mark this point within the tender area.

Technique

Insert the needle into the centre of the tender area, over the superolateral aspect of the greater trochanter, until the needle rests between the insertion of gluteus maximus into the iliotibial tract, and the underlying greater trochanter (Figs 8.5 and 8.6). This usually reproduces the patient's pain. Deliver the injection by a bolus technique if no resistance is felt, or if this is not possible a peppering technique, aiming to cover the full extent of the tender area within the bursa.

Patient advice

Advise the patient to maintain a period of relative rest for up to 2 weeks after the injection.

Causative factors should be addressed to prevent recurrence. It may be appropriate to introduce a regime of stretching techniques for the iliotibial tract.

▶ **FIGURE 8.5**

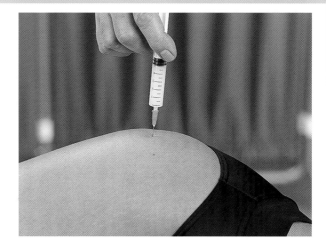

▶ **FIGURE 8.6**

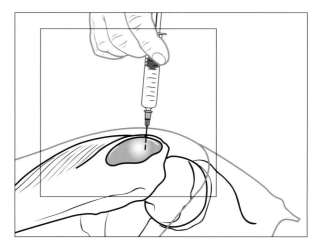

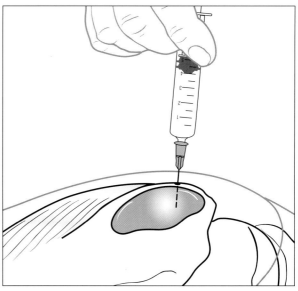

ORIGIN OF THE HAMSTRINGS AT THE ISCHIAL TUBEROSITY

Indication

Hamstring tendinitis (enthesitis). The hamstring muscles are commonly strained during sporting activities. As two joint muscles, they act to extend the hip and flex the knee and are relatively weak in comparison to the quadriceps (Sutton 1984). The ballistic action of sprinting commonly leads to acute lesions in the muscle bellies, while overuse activities are more likely to produce strain of the common origin at the ischial tuberosity.

Patient presentation

The patient complains of a gradual onset of pain in the lower buttock area, localized to the ischial tuberosity.

On examination, pain is reproduced on testing resisted knee flexion and on passively testing the straight-leg raise.

Treatment by injection

Injection into the common origin of the hamstrings at the ischial tuberosity (the enthesis) may be curative for chronic strain. Alternative treatment modalities may be considered, such as mobilization by deep transverse friction massage and electrotherapy.

Needle size	23 G × 1 in (0.6 × 25 mm) blue needle (or larger if more appropriate for the patient).

Dose	20 mg triamcinolone acetonide, 1 ml local anaesthetic, e.g. 0.5 ml Kenalog®, 1 ml 1% lidocaine.

Patient position

Position the patient in side lying, with the hip and knee flexed to a right angle.

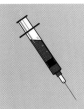

ALTERNATIVE TECHNIQUE: Position the patient in prone lying over the side edge of a plinth, with the hip and knee flexed to a right angle. The knee should be supported on a stool.

Palpation

The positions described above expose the ischial tuberosity from under the gluteus maximus muscle. Locate the area of tenderness in the tendon, commonly found at its teno-osseous junction on the ischial tuberosity, and mark this point.

Technique

Insert the needle perpendicular to the tendon and ischial tuberosity and deliver the injection by a peppering technique (Figs 8.7 and 8.8).

Patient advice

Advise the patient to maintain a period of relative rest for up to 2 weeks following injection. It is important to establish an appropriate training regime for full rehabilitation of the hamstrings, and the causative factors of any overuse injury should be addressed.

▶ **FIGURE 8.7**

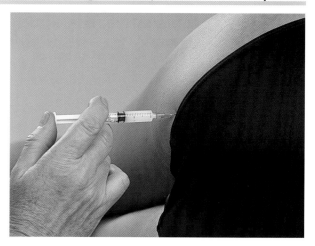

▶ **FIGURE 8.8**

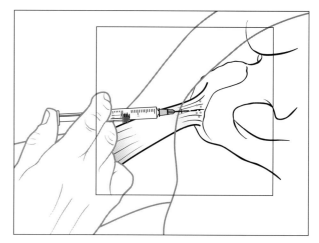

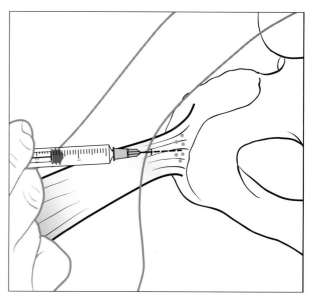

ORIGIN OF ADDUCTOR LONGUS

Indication

Adductor tendinitis (enthesitis). Strain of the adductor longus tendon, commonly known as 'rider's strain'. Overuse of the adductors, e.g. while working a horse, may produce chronic tendinitis. A single traumatic incident, in which the tendon is overstretched, may be the cause of an acute lesion.

Patient presentation

The patient complains of pain localized to the groin area or referred to the medial aspect of the thigh.

On examination, the symptoms will be reproduced by resisted adduction and on stretching, by passive abduction.

Treatment by injection

An injection at the teno-osseous junction of the origin of adductor longus with the body of the pubis (the enthesis) may be curative. Alternative physiotherapeutic modalities may also be considered.

Needle size	23 G × 1¼ in (0.6 × 30 mm) blue needle.

Dose	20 mg triamcinolone acetonide, 1 ml local anaesthetic, e.g. 0.5 ml Kenalog®, 1 ml 1% lidocaine.

Patient position

Position the patient in supine lying on a plinth, with the leg supported in a degree of abduction and lateral rotation.

Palpation

Locate the area of tenderness at the teno-osseous junction on the body of the pubis, in the angle between the crest and the symphysis pubis. Mark this area.

Technique

Insert the needle just distal to the teno-osseous junction, angling obliquely upwards toward the body of the pubis (Figs 8.9 and 8.10). Deliver the

▶ FIGURE 8.9

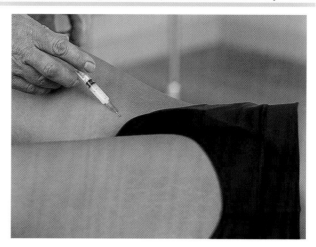

▶ FIGURE 8.10

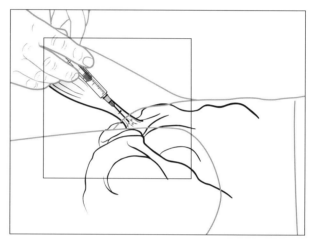

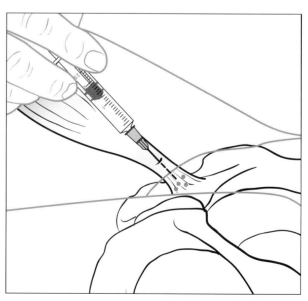

injection by a peppering technique, covering the full extent of the lesion as identified by palpation.

Patient advice

Advise the patient to maintain a period of relative rest for up to 2 weeks following the injection. Once the symptoms and signs have subsided, a full rehabilitation programme can be followed, including stretching if necessary.

9 The knee

KNEE JOINT

Indication

Arthritis, which may be due to an acute episode of degenerative osteoarthrosis or inflammatory arthritis. Traumatic arthritis is usually a secondary response to a ligamentous lesion at the knee and should be treated as such (*see* Kesson & Atkins 1998).

Patient presentation

The patient may complain of a gradual or sudden onset of pain and swelling at the knee. The pain may be anterior and/or posterior since the knee lies within the L3/4 and S1/2 dermatomes. Symptoms are generally aggravated by weight-bearing activities and the knee may be stiff after rest.

On examination, swelling and synovial thickening may be palpated. A capsular pattern of greater limitation of flexion than extension is present and flexion has a harder than normal end-feel.

Needle size	21 G × 1$^1/_2$ in (0.8 × 40 mm) green needle.

Dose	30 mg triamcinolone acetonide, 1 ml local anaesthetic, e.g. 3 ml Adcortyl®, 1 ml 1% lidocaine.

Treatment by injection

An intra-articular injection of corticosteroid may be beneficial in the treatment of symptomatic osteoarthrosis or inflammatory arthritis (Dieppe et al 1980). The possible mechanical causes of traumatic arthritis (e.g. ligamentous lesion) should be addressed directly.

Patient position

Position the patient in half lying and support the knee in the extended position.

Palpation

Palpate the patella and glide it medially, pressing down on the lateral border to lift the medial edge. Mark a point at the approximate mid-point of the medial border of the patella.

Technique

Insert the needle at the mid-point of the medial border of the patella, angling laterally and slightly posteriorly to allow for the convex shape of the posterior surface of the patella (Figs 9.1 and 9.2). Once intracapsular, and when there is no resistance to the injection, deliver by a bolus technique.

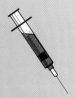

ALTERNATIVE TECHNIQUES:

1. Glide the patella laterally. Insert the needle at the mid-point of the lateral border of the patella, aiming medially and slightly posteriorly with the needle parallel to the articular surface of the patella. Deliver by a bolus technique.
2. If a visible effusion is present, the needle may be inserted into the suprapatellar pouch and intra-articular placement confirmed by initial aspiration before injecting as a bolus.
3. Position the patient supine or half lying, with the knee flexed. Insert the needle below the apex of the patella on either the medial or the lateral side of the patellar tendon (in acupuncture, the 'eyes' of the knee) and once intracapsular, deliver as a bolus.
4. Sambrook et al (1989) noted that much of the pain of degenerative arthritis of the knee is due to abnormal stress on the extensor mechanism, including the capsular attachments to the patellar margins. Peripatellar infiltration of corticosteroid was demonstrated to be at least as useful as the standard intra-articular injection technique.

▶ FIGURE 9.1

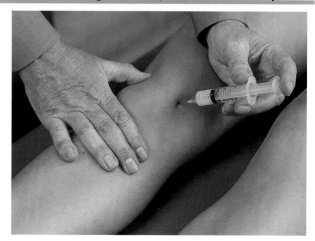

▶ FIGURE 9.2

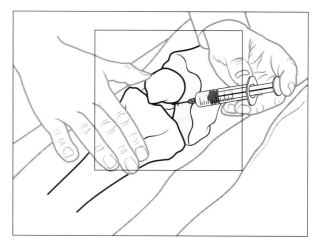

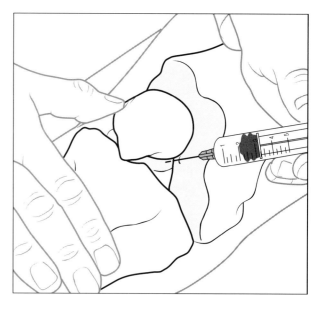

CLINICAL TIP: There is some controversy concerning repeated steroid injections into weight-bearing joints and the associated risk of developing steroid arthropathy (Parikh et al 1993, Cameron 1995a). To minimize risk of steroid arthropathy, it is recommended that weight-bearing joints should not be injected more frequently than every 4–6 months.

Patient advice

Advise the patent to maintain a period of relative rest for up to 2 weeks after the injection. Chakravarty and Pharoah (1994) showed that 24 hours of complete bed-rest following injection of the knee joint for rheumatoid arthritis produced more prolonged benefit.

BAKER'S CYST

This is a fluctuant swelling which appears on the posterior aspect of the knee joint line. It is associated with pathology in the knee joint such as degenerative or inflammatory arthritis and treatment should be directed at the knee joint itself.

BURSITIS ASSOCIATED WITH THE PATELLA

Indication

Prepatellar bursitis (housemaid's knee) and **superficial infrapatellar bursitis** (clergyman's knee), which are usually associated with friction between the patella or patellar tendon and the skin. Since these are subcutaneous bursae they are vulnerable to unrecognized perforating injuries, therefore it is important that the patient is screened for possible infection before injecting with corticosteroid.

Patient presentation

The patient complains of a gradual onset of aching pain felt superficial to the patella or patellar tendon, depending on which bursa is involved.

On examination, there are usually no clinical findings except for the obvious swelling over the patella.

Needle size	21 G × $1\frac{1}{2}$ in (0.8 × 40 mm) green needle.

Dose	10 mg triamcinolone acetonide, 1 ml local anaesthetic, e.g. 1 ml Adcortyl®, 1 ml 1% lidocaine.

Treatment by injection

An injection into the bursa can be curative.

Patient position

Position the patient in half lying and support the knee in the extended position.

Palpation

Palpate the tender, swollen area of the bursa on the anterior aspect of the patella or patellar tendon and mark a central point convenient for the injection.

Technique

Insert the needle at the mid-point of the tender area and inject as a bolus when the bursa is identified by a loss of resistance to the needle insertion (Figs 9.3 and 9.4).

Patient advice

The patient should be advised to avoid further trauma to the bursa.

▶ **FIGURE 9.3**

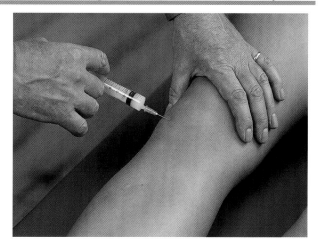

▶ **FIGURE 9.4**

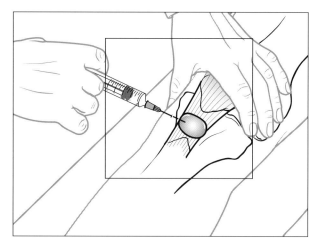

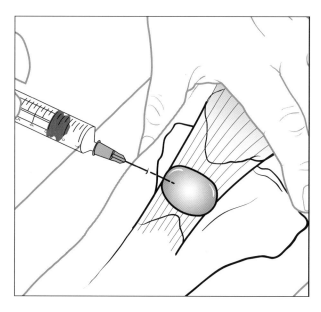

PES ANSERINE BURSA

Indication

Bursitis, commonly due to overuse (Hutson 1990). This bursa is located on the medial aspect of the knee deep to the pes anserine ('goose's foot') tendon, that comprises the tendons of sartorius, gracilis and semitendinosus.

Patient presentation

The patient may complain of a gradual onset of aching pain felt on the medial aspect of the knee.

On examination, passive movements and resisted tests are generally negative, but swelling and tenderness to palpation are present on the anteromedial aspect of the tibia just below the joint line.

Needle size	23 G × 1 in (0.6 × 25 mm) blue needle or 25 G × $^5/_8$ in (0.5 × 16 mm) orange needle.

Dose	20 mg triamcinolone acetonide, 1 ml local anaesthetic, e.g. 0.5 ml Kenalog®, 1 ml 1% lidocaine.

Treatment by injection

An injection into the bursa can be curative.

Patient position

Position the patient half-lying and support the knee in the extended position.

Palpation

Palpate the tender, swollen area of the bursa on the medial aspect of the tibia and mark a central point convenient for the injection.

Technique

Insert the needle at the mid-point of the tender area and inject as a bolus when the bursa is identified by a loss of resistance to the needle insertion (Figs 9.5 and 9.6).

Patient advice

The patient should be advised to avoid further trauma to the bursa.

▶ FIGURE 9.5

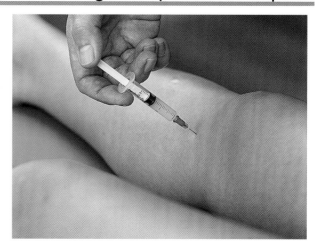

▶ FIGURE 9.6

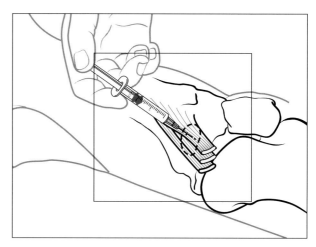

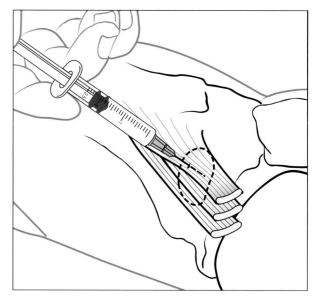

CORONARY LIGAMENTS

Indication

Sprain of the coronary ligaments due to a rotational or hyperextension injury at the knee. The coronary (meniscotibial) ligaments attach the menisci to the upper surface of the tibia. The longer lateral coronary ligaments are less commonly involved, but the shorter medial coronary ligaments are vulnerable to sprain, especially in association with medial meniscal damage.

Discussion here is of the more commonly affected medial coronary ligaments, but if the lateral coronary ligaments were involved, the same principles would apply.

Patient presentation

The patient complains of pain on the medial aspect of the knee, possibly related to a rotational or hyperextension injury. On examination there is a non-capsular pattern of pain on passive lateral rotation of the knee.

Treatment by injection

This lesion responds very well to physiotherapeutic modalities, transverse friction massage in particular (Cyriax & Cyriax 1983, Cyriax 1984, Kesson & Atkins 1998). In more chronic cases, an injection may also be curative and is an alternative treatment to physiotherapy.

Needle size	23 G × 1 in (0.6 × 25mm) blue needle.

Dose	10 mg triamcinolone acetonide, 0.75 ml local anaesthetic, e.g. 0.25 ml Kenalog®, 0.75 ml 1% lidocaine.

Patient position

Position the patient lying with the knee flexed and laterally rotated to expose the medial tibial condyle.

Palpation

Palpate the superior surface of the medial tibial plateau for the area of tenderness in the medial coronary ligaments. Mark the area of tenderness.

Technique

Insert the needle tangentially to the meniscus and deliver the injection by peppering technique along the affected area of the ligament (Figs 9.7 and 9.8).

Patient advice

Advise the patient to maintain a period of relative rest for up to 2 weeks after the injection.

▶ **FIGURE 9.7**

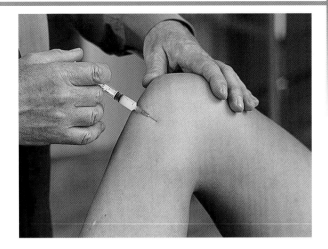

▶ **FIGURE 9.8**

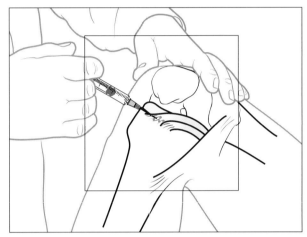

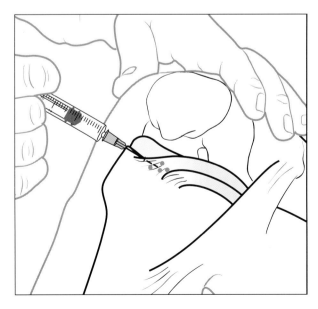

INFRAPATELLAR TENDON

Indication

Infrapatellar tendinitis ('jumper's knee'), which may be due to repetitive overuse, particularly arising from activities that involve a jumping action, resulting in microfailure and fraying of the tendon fibres with areas of focal degeneration (Curwin & Stanish 1984).

Patient presentation

The patient complains of a gradual onset of anterior knee pain, usually localized to the inferior pole of the patella.

On examination, the pain is reproduced at the front of the knee by resisted knee extension.

Treatment by injection

An injection into the teno-osseous junction of the infrapatellar tendon may be curative, but the cause of the lesion should also be addressed to prevent recurrence.

Needle size	23 G × 1 in (0.6 × 25 mm) blue needle.

Dose	20 mg triamcinolone acetonide, 1 ml local anaesthetic, e.g. 0.5 ml Kenalog®, 1 ml 1% lidocaine.

Patient position

Position the patient in half lying, with the knee supported in extension.

Palpation

Tilt the inferior pole (apex) of the patella upward by applying downward pressure over the superior pole (base) with the web space between your index finger and thumb. Palpate the teno-osseous junction of the infrapatellar tendon and mark the area of tenderness.

Technique

Insert the needle just distal to the inferior pole of the patella, at the mid-point of the area of tenderness, angling upward to make contact with the bone at the teno-osseous junction of the tendon (Figs 9.9 and 9.10). Fanning outwards from this mid-position, deliver the injection by peppering technique, depositing two parallel rows of droplets of solution along the affected part of the teno-osseous junction.

CLINICAL TIP: To avoid weakening of the collagen fibre content of this weight-bearing tendon, the injection is **NOT** delivered into the body of the tendon but at the teno-osseous junction.

Patient advice

Advise the patient to maintain a period of relative rest from all aggravating and overuse factors for up to 2 weeks following the injection.

Alternative treatments for infrapatellar tendinitis may include physiotherapeutic modalities such as mobilization by transverse friction massage (Cyriax & Cyriax 1983, Cyriax 1984, Kesson & Atkins 1998). The condition may be due to maltracking mechanisms of the patella and this may need to be addressed by corrective taping techniques and specific exercises.

▶ FIGURE 9.9

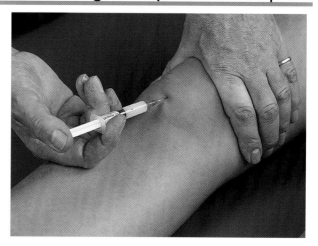

▶ FIGURE 9.10

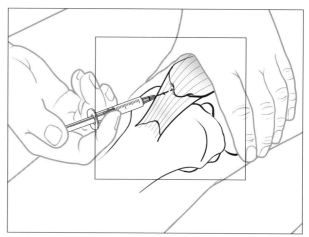

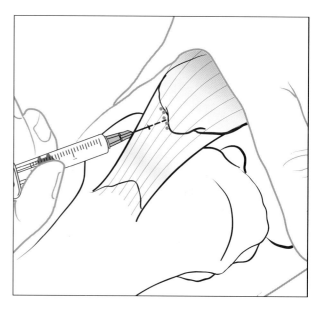

SUPRAPATELLAR TENDON

Indication

Suprapatellar tendinitis, which is not as common as infrapatellar tendinitis, but the cause, disease process and management, are the same (*see* p. 140).

Patient presentation

The patient complains of a gradual onset of pain felt at the superior pole (base) of the patella.

On examination, the pain is reproduced at the front of the knee by resisted knee extension.

Treatment by injection

An injection into the teno-osseous junction of the suprapatellar tendon may be curative, but the cause of the lesion should also be addressed to prevent recurrence.

Needle size	23 G × 1 in (0.6 × 25 mm) blue needle.

Dose	20 mg triamcinolone acetonide, 1 ml local anaesthetic, e.g. 0.5 ml Kenalog®, 1 ml 1% lidocaine.

Patient position

Position the patient in half lying, with the knee supported in extension.

Palpation

Tilt the superior pole (base) of the patella upward by applying downward pressure over the inferior pole (apex) with the web space between your index finger and thumb. Palpate the teno-osseous junction of the suprapatellar tendon and mark the area of tenderness.

Technique

Insert the needle just proximal to the superior pole of the patella, at the mid-point of the area of tenderness, angling downward to make contact with the bone at the teno-osseous junction of the tendon (Figs 9.11 and 9.12). Fanning outwards from this mid-position, deliver the injection by a peppering technique, depositing two parallel rows of droplets of solution along the affected part of the teno-osseous junction.

Patient advice

Advise the patient to maintain a period of relative rest for up to 2 weeks after the injection.

Alternatively, treatment for suprapatellar tendinitis may be by physio-therapeutic modalities including mobilization by transverse friction massage (Cyriax & Cyriax 1983, Cyriax 1984, Kesson & Atkins 1998). The condition may be due to maltracking mechanisms of the patella and this may need to be addressed by corrective taping techniques and specific exercises.

▶ **FIGURE 9.11**

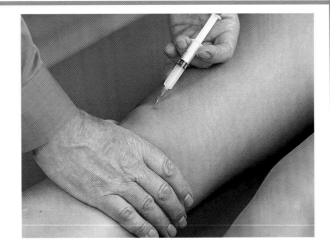

▶ **FIGURE 9.12**

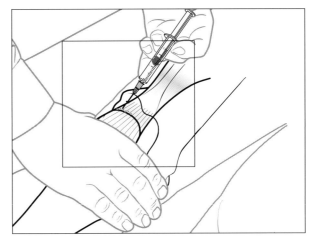

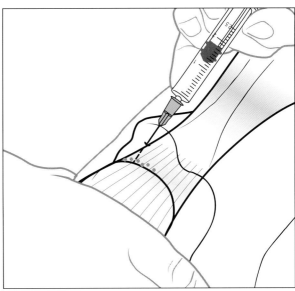

10 The ankle and foot

ANKLE (TALOCRURAL) JOINT

Indication

Arthritis, which may be an acute episode of degenerative osteoarthrosis, inflammatory arthritis, such as rheumatoid arthritis, or traumatic arthritis associated with fracture or ligamentous injury. Degenerative osteoarthrosis in this joint is not common unless there has been a precipitating cause such as fracture, instability or postural overuse.

Patient presentation

The patient complains of pain and swelling located locally around the ankle joint.

On examination, a capsular pattern of limited movement will be evident, with a greater limitation of plantarflexion than dorsiflexion. Plantarflexion will exhibit an abnormal hard end-feel.

Treatment by injection

An intra-articular injection may reduce the pain and swelling, allowing an increase in the range of mobility at the ankle joint.

| **Needle size** | 23 G × 1 in (0.6 × 25 mm) blue needle or 21 G × 1½ in (0.8 × 40 mm) green needle. |

Dose	20 mg triamcinolone acetonide, 1 ml local anaesthetic, e.g. 2 ml Adcortyl®, 1 ml 1% lidocaine.

Patient position

Position the patient in half lying, with the knee flexed and the foot flat on the plinth. This places the ankle in a degree of plantarflexion, which opens the anterior aspect of the joint.

Palpation

Palpate the anterior ankle joint line to locate a suitable entry point into the ankle joint. Generally this will be between the tendons of tibialis anterior and extensor hallucis longus, but a point of entry may also be made at the upper, inner aspect of either malleolus. Mark the selected point of entry on the joint line.

CLINICAL TIP: The dorsalis pedis artery and deep peroneal nerve lie just lateral to the extensor hallucis longus tendon at the ankle joint. These structures should be avoided when selecting the point for needle insertion.

Technique

Insert the needle at the point marked anteriorly and angle the needle upward to run parallel to the upper surface of the talus, which is slightly convex (Figs 10.1 and 10.2). Once the needle is intracapsular, deliver the injection as a bolus.

CLINICAL TIP: There is some controversy concerning repeated steroid injections into weight-bearing joints and the associated risk of developing steroid arthropathy (Parikh et al 1993, Cameron 1995a). To minimize risk of steroid arthropathy, it is recommended that weight-bearing joints should not be injected more frequently than every 4–6 months.

Patient advice

Advise the patient to maintain a period of relative rest for up to 2 weeks after the injection.

▶ **FIGURE 10.1**

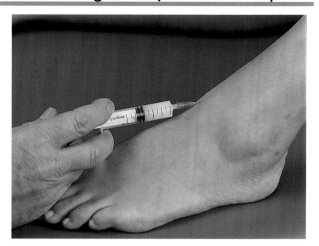

▶ **FIGURE 10.2**

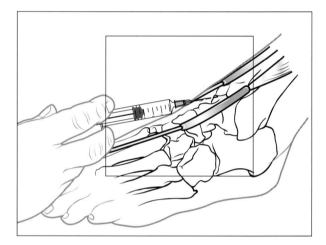

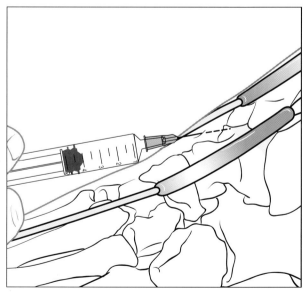

SUBTALAR (TALOCALCANEAL) JOINT

Indication

Arthritis, the commonest form being inflammatory rheumatoid arthritis.

Patient presentation

The patient complains of pain and swelling in the ankle region.

On examination, a capsular pattern of limited movement is present, i.e. limitation of supination, and in advanced cases the hind foot fixes in pronation.

Treatment by injection

Corticosteroid injection may alleviate the symptoms.

Needle size	23 G × 1 in (0.6 × 25 mm) blue needle.

Dose	10 mg triamcinolone acetonide, 1 ml local anaesthetic, e.g. 1 ml Adcortyl®, 1 ml 1% lidocaine.

Patient position

Position the patient in half lying, with the lower leg supported.

Palpation

Locate the subtalar joint by palpating the sustentaculum tali of the calcaneum, which lies approximately one thumb's width directly below the medial malleolus. Just above this bony, horizontal ridge lies the subtalar joint line. This joint is wider posteriorly and more easily entered there. Mark this point.

Technique

The anatomy of the subtalar joint is complicated, as the joint is divided into two compartments by an interosseous ligament. Insert the needle into the point marked (see above) and first angle it posteriorly, to deliver approximately half of the corticosteroid solution into the posterior compartment as a bolus

(Figs 10.3 and 10.4). Withdrawing the needle slightly, but not out through the skin, reposition it anteriorly and deliver the remainder of the solution into the anterior compartment (Figs 10.5 and 10.6), also as a bolus.

CLINICAL TIP: The posterior tibial artery and tibial nerve lie below and behind the sustentaculum tali. Locate the tibial artery pulse by palpation. Avoid these structures by accurately selecting the needle insertion point as indicated and by angling the needle as described.

ALTERNATIVE TECHNIQUE: Insert the needle laterally via the sinus tarsi, which is located by palpation antero-inferiorly to the lateral malleolus. Deliver by a bolus technique.

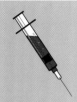

CLINICAL TIP: There is some controversy concerning repeated steroid injections into weight-bearing joints and the associated risk of developing steroid arthropathy (Parikh et al 1993, Cameron 1995a). To minimize risk of steroid arthropathy, it is recommended that weight-bearing joints should not be injected more frequently than every 4–6 months.

Patient advice

Advise the patient to maintain a period of relative rest for up to 2 weeks following the injection.

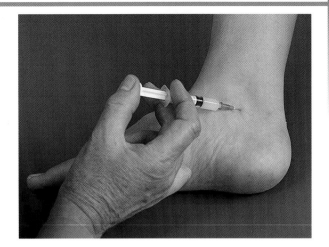

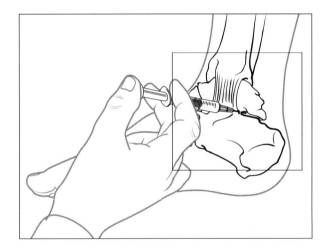

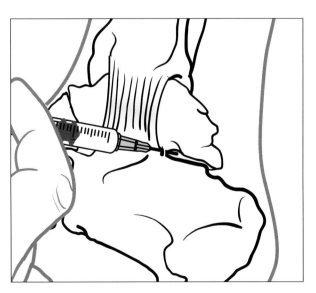

▶ **FIGURE 10.5**

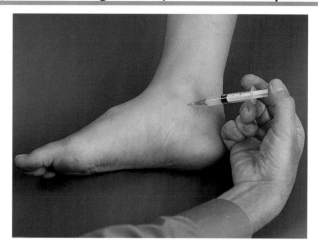

▶ **FIGURE 10.6**

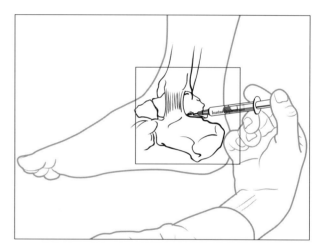

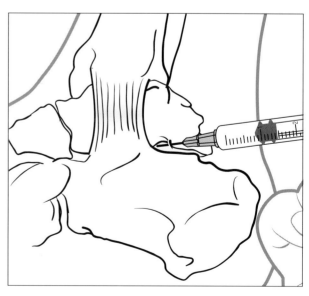

MID-TARSAL (TRANSVERSE TARSAL) JOINT

Indication

Arthritis, which may be acute episodes of degenerative osteoarthritis, inflammatory arthritis or traumatic arthritis.

Patient presentation

The patient complains of pain and swelling felt over the mid-foot region.

On examination, the capsular pattern of limited movement will be present, with limitation of adduction and supination. In advanced cases the foot fixes in abduction and pronation.

Treatment by injection

Symptomatic relief can be gained from an intra-articular injection of corticosteroid.

Needle size	23 G × 1 in (0.6 × 25 mm) blue needle.

Dose	10 mg triamcinolone acetonide, 0.5 ml local anaesthetic, e.g. 1 ml Adcortyl®, 0.5 ml 1% lidocaine.

Patient position

Position the patient comfortably supported in half lying.

Palpation

The midtarsal complex consists of the calcaneocuboid joint laterally and the talocalcaneonavicular joint medially. Palpate the joints to identify the site of the lesion. The calcaneocuboid joint is located approximately one thumb's width behind and above the base of the fifth metatarsal. The talocalcaneonavicular joint is located by passively everting the foot and palpating along the talus in front of the medial malleolus until the joint line is felt. Mark the selected point of entry over the appropriate joint line.

Technique

Insert the needle perpendicular to the joint line and, once intracapsular, deliver the injection as a bolus (Figs 10.7 & 10.8).

CLINICAL TIP: The dorsalis pedis artery and deep peroneal nerve lie on the dorsum of the foot lateral to the extensor hallucis longus tendon. Locate the dorsalis pedis pulse by palpation and avoid injecting into the artery or nerve by considering their positions in the foot.

Patient advice

Advise the patient to maintain a period or relative rest for up to 2 weeks after the injection.

▶ FIGURE 10.7

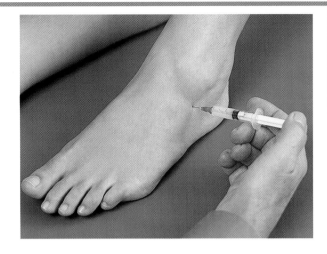

▶ FIGURE 10.8

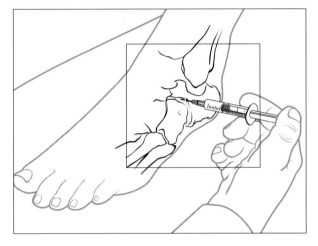

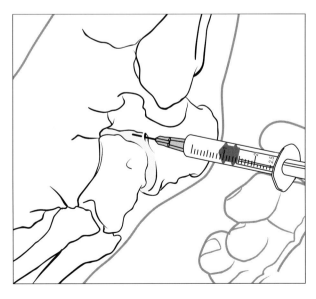

FIRST METATARSOPHALANGEAL JOINT

Indication

Arthritis, which may be an acute episode of degenerative osteoarthrosis, inflammatory arthritis or traumatic arthritis.

Patient presentation

The patient complains of pain, and often swelling, located locally over the big toe.

On examination, a capsular pattern of limited movement will be present with gross loss of extension and some loss of flexion. The loss of extension can hamper function, since it is required for the toe-off phase of gait.

Treatment by injection

An injection of corticosteroid can give good symptomatic relief and allow mobilization to restore the range of movement.

Needle size	25 G × ⁵/₈ in (0.5 × 16 mm) orange needle.

Dose	10 mg triamcinolone acetonide, 0.25 ml local anaesthetic, e.g. 0.25 ml Kenalog®, 0.25 ml 1% lidocaine.

Patient position

Position the patient in half lying, with the foot supported.

Palpation

The joint line is located dorsally by palpation, but if this is difficult add some distraction, which will also facilitate the injection. Mark a point on the joint line, selecting either side of the extensor tendon.

Technique

Insert the needle perpendicular to the joint line and, once intracapsular, deliver the injection as a bolus (Figs 10.9 and 10.10).

Patient advice

Advise the patient to maintain a period of relative rest for up to two weeks after the injection.

▶ **FIGURE 10.9**

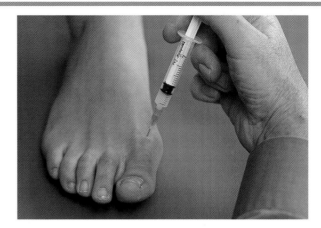

▶ **FIGURE 10.10**

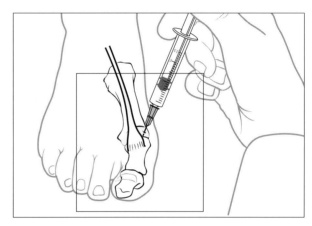

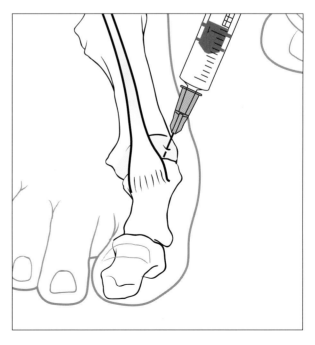

METATARSOPHALANGEAL AND INTERPHALANGEAL JOINTS

Indication

Arthritis. Degenerative, inflammatory or traumatic arthritis may affect these joints.

Patient presentation

The patient will be able to localize their pain to the particular joint(s) involved.

On examination, the capsular pattern of limited movement will confirm the diagnosis. This pattern may vary, but generally there is a greater limitation of flexion at the metatarsophalangeal joints causing them to fix in extension, while the interphalangeal joints fix in flexion.

Treatment by injection

Corticosteroid injection reduces the inflammation and may achieve effective pain relief.

Needle size	25 G × $^5/_8$ in (0.5 × 16 mm) orange needle.

Dose	10 mg triamcinolone acetonide, 0.25 ml local anaesthetic, e.g. 0.25 ml Kenalog®, 0.25 ml 1% lidocaine.

Patient position

Position the patient in half lying, with the foot supported.

Palpation

Locate the symptomatic joint and identify the joint line. Mark a point on the dorsolateral or dorsomedial joint line.

Technique

Insert the needle perpendicularly into the relevant joint, via the dorsolateral or dorsomedial surface to avoid the extensor tendon (Figs 10.11 and 10.12). Once intracapsular, the injection can be delivered as a bolus.

Patient advice

Advise the patient to maintain a period of relative rest for up to 2 weeks after the injection.

▶ **FIGURE 10.11**

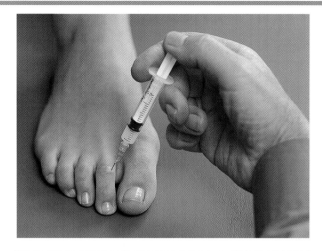

▶ **FIGURE 10.12**

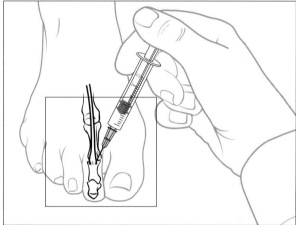

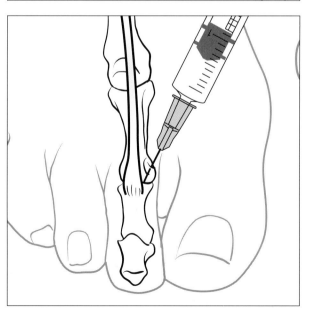

SESAMOIDITIS

Indication

Bruising of the sesamoid bone of flexor hallucis longus or traumatic arthritis of the sesamo-first-metatarsal joint associated with deformity such as pes cavus (Cyriax 1982).

Patient presentation

The patient complains of pain on the medial aspect of the plantar surface of the forefoot on walking. On examination, pain may be provoked by resisted flexion of the big toe and there is an area of tenderness to palpation.

Treatment by injection

Injection may be curative (Cyriax 1982).

Needle size	23 G × 1 in (0.6 × 25mm) blue needle.

Dose	10 mg triamcinolone acetonide, 0.75 ml local anaesthetic, e.g. 0.25 ml Kenalog®, 0.75 ml 1% lidocaine.

Patient position

Position the patient comfortably sitting or lying, with the foot supported.

Palpation

Palpate and mark the area of tenderness on the plantar aspect of the big toe.

Technique

Insert the needle medially on the plantar surface of the big toe, aiming towards the area of tenderness between the first metatarsal and the flexor tendon (Figs 10.13 and 10.14). Deliver the injection by a bolus technique, avoiding direct injection into the tendon.

CLINICAL TIP: The digital arteries and nerves run alongside the flexor tendons and need to be considered when administering the injection.

▶ FIGURE 10.13

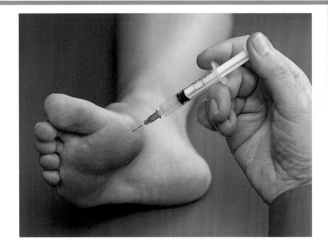

▶ FIGURE 10.14

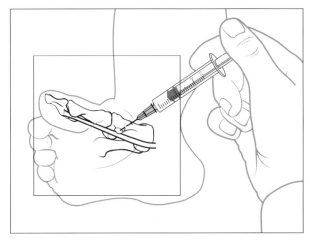

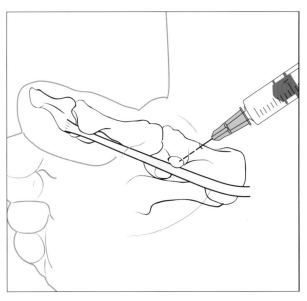

RETROCALCANEAL BURSA

Indication

Retrocalcaneal bursitis, which may be due to the existence of a bony exostosis (Haglund's deformity), or ill-fitting footwear which exerts excessive pressure over the posterior aspect of the heel. The condition may be a manifestation of rheumatoid arthritis or one of the spondyloarthropathies, e.g. Reiter's disease (Hutson 1990, Frey et al 1992, Baxter 1994).

Patient presentation

The patient complains of pain felt on the posterior aspect of the heel. Aggravating factors include sporting activities and footwear.

On examination, the signs may be confusing and it may be difficult to differentiate the condition from Achilles tendinitis, with which it may co-exist. Passive dorsiflexion, passive plantarflexion and resisted plantarflexion may all squeeze the inflamed bursa, but palpation just anterior and to either side of the Achilles tendon will localize the lesion.

Treatment by injection

An injection of corticosteroid may give symptomatic relief of pain, but the cause of the problem must be addressed to prevent recurrence.

Needle size	23 G × 1 in (0.6 × 25 mm) blue needle.

Dose	10 mg triamcinolone acetonide, 0.5 ml local anaesthetic, e.g. 0.25 ml Kenalog®, 0.5 ml 1% lidocaine.

Patient position

Position the patient in prone lying, with the foot supported in slight plantarflexion over a pillow. Supine lying could also be used.

Palpation

Frey et al (1992) used X-ray and contrast medium to demonstrate the existence of the retrocalcaneal bursa. It caps the superoposterior surface of the calcaneum as a horseshoe-shaped bursa, separating the calcaneum from the insertion of the Achilles tendon (Stephens 1994). The tender bursa can be located by palpation anterior to the tendon, either laterally or medially to the distal end of the Achilles tendon. Mark the identified point of maximum tenderness.

Technique

Insert the needle either medially or laterally between the distal end of the Achilles tendon and the upper third of the posterior surface of the calcaneum (Figs 10.15 and 10.16). Deliver the injection as a bolus.

Patient advice

Advise the patient to maintain a period of relative rest for up to 2 weeks following the injection. The cause of the condition should be addressed by avoiding aggravating activities or replacing ill-fitting footwear.

▶ FIGURE 10.15

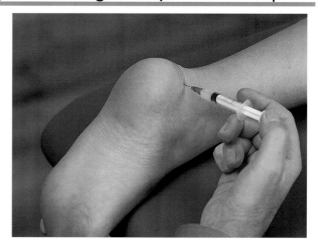

▶ FIGURE 10.16

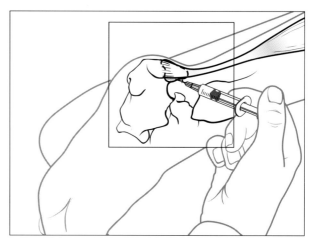

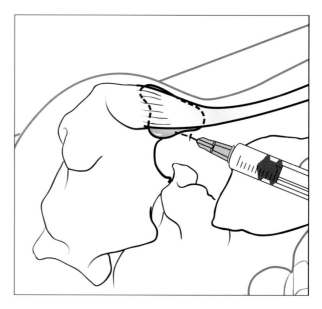

'DANCER'S HEEL'

Indication

Posterior tibial periostitis, which may occur particularly in ballet dancers, where the increased mobility into plantarflexion at the ankle joint resulting from point work causes the calcaneum to bruise the periosteum at the lower border of the posterior tibia (Cyriax 1982). A similar condition can be seen in other athletes, e.g. footballers, javelin throwers, hockey and squash players (Cyriax & Cyriax 1983).

Patient presentation

The patient complains of pain felt locally at the back of the heel, with symptoms reproduced at the end of range of passive plantarflexion (Cyriax 1982).

Treatment by injection

Injection may be curative providing the cause of the lesion is addressed.

Needle size	21 G × 1½ in (0.8 × 40 mm) or 21 G × 2 in (0.8 × 50 mm) green needle.

Dose	10 mg triamcinolone acetonide, 0.75 ml local anaesthetic, e.g. 0.25 ml Kenalog®, 0.75 ml 1% lidocaine.

Patient position

Position the patient in prone lying.

Palpation

Palpate and mark the area of tenderness on the posterior aspect of the lower tibia deep to the Achilles tendon.

Technique

Insert the needle either medially or laterally to the Achilles tendon, aiming towards the posterior margin of the lower tibia which lies approximately 2 cm above a line joining the malleoli, and deliver the injection by a peppering technique across the periosteum of the lower edge of the tibia (Figs 10.17 and 10.18).

Patient advice

Advise the patient to maintain a period of relative rest for up to two weeks following the injection. The patient should be made aware of the causative factors and measures should be taken to avoid over pointing.

▶ **FIGURE 10.17**

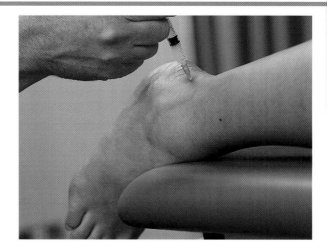

▶ **FIGURE 10.18**

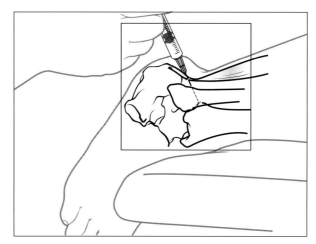

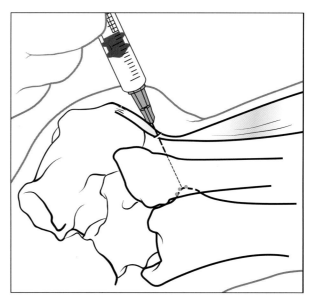

PLANTAR FASCIA

Indication

Plantar fasciitis, which may be due to repetitive microtrauma of the longitudinal arch of the foot, producing focal tears and chronic inflammation at the insertion of the plantar fascia into the medial tuberosity of the calcaneum (Kibler et al 1991, Karr 1994, Gibbon & Cassar-Pullicino 1994, Dasgupta & Bowles 1995, Singh et al 1997). Repeated intrinsic muscle activity against the stretched plantar fascia during gait activities may cause a traction injury of the plantar fascia at its insertion (Gibbon & Cassar-Pullicino 1994). Both of these mechanisms may produce a heel spur. Obesity can be a predisposing factor, since it may lead to postural overuse of the foot, causing overpronation and stretching of the plantar fascia. A tight Achilles tendon may also produce overpronation, and inappropriate footwear may predispose to the condition (Evans 1990, Karr 1994).

Patient presentation

The patient complains of a gradual onset of pain on the medial aspect of the plantar surface of the heel. Characteristically, this is most painful when the first few steps are taken as the patient gets out of bed in the morning, but the pain then eases (Kibler et al 1991, Karr 1994).

On examination, positive signs may be lacking on routine examination of the foot and ankle. Passive extension of the toes may have a 'windlass' effect on the plantar fascia, reproducing the pain. Exquisite tenderness is present specifically over the medial calcaneal tuberosity.

Treatment by injection

A corticosteroid injection can be curative. Sellman (1994) suggested that an accurate injection abolishes pain and tenderness, preventing the need for repeated injections which have been associated with plantar fascia rupture. Singh et al (1997) suggests a comprehensive treatment programme, including corticosteroid injection, intrinsic muscle exercises, calf stretches, strapping and heel cushions, and 'cock-up' night splints may be needed to address the problem.

Needle size	21 G × 1¹/₂ in (0.8 × 40 mm) or 21 G × 2 in (0.8 × 50 mm) green needle.

Dose	20 mg triamcinolone acetonide, 1 ml local anaesthetic, e.g. 0.5 ml Kenalog®, 1 ml 1% lidocaine.

Patient position

Position the patient in prone lying, with the knee slightly flexed and the lower leg supported on a pillow. The position can be modified to allow the patient to lie supine.

Palpation

Locate the medial calcaneal tuberosity by deep palpation and mark the mid-point of the tender area.

Technique

Insert the needle through the soft tissues on the medial aspect of the foot anterior to the marked point (Fig. 10.19). Angle the needle posterolaterally towards the junction of the plantar fascia with the medial calcaneal tuberosity (Fig. 10.20), and deliver the injection by peppering technique. This indirect approach to the plantar fascia is more comfortable for the patient, since the needle is inserted through soft tissue, rather than directly through the fat pad. It also avoids fat atrophy and the risk of infection from the sole of the foot.

CLINICAL TIP: The lateral plantar artery and nerve and the medial plantar nerves lie deep to the origin of the plantar fascia.

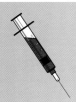

ALTERNATIVE TECHNIQUES: Position as above:

1. Insert the needle perpendicular to the sole of the foot aiming towards the area of tenderness where the injection is delivered by a peppering technique.
2. Insert the needle medially, perpendicular to the calcaneum, aiming towards the area of tenderness where the injection is delivered by a peppering technique.

Patient advice

Advise the patient to maintain a period of relative rest for up to 2 weeks after the injection. The causative factors should be addressed to prevent recurrence, including weight loss if appropriate.

▶ **FIGURE 10.19**

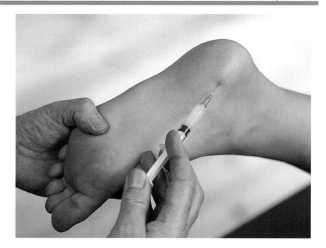

▶ **FIGURE 10.20**

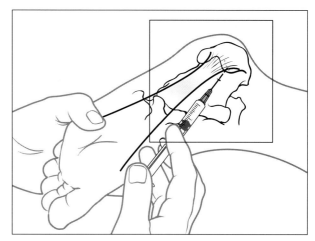

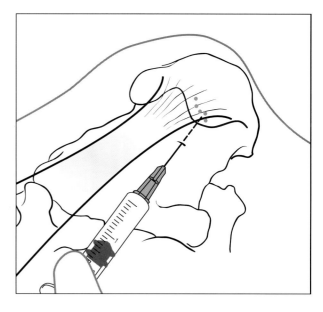

PERONEAL TENDONS

Indication

Tendinitis at the teno-osseous junction of peroneus brevis at the base of the fifth metatarsal, or **tenosynovitis** of peroneus longus and brevis in their shared synovial sheath at the ankle. An acute lesion may be associated with inversion sprain at the ankle; the chronic lesion may be due to overuse.

Patient presentation

The patient complains of either sudden pain felt on the lateral side of the ankle following an inversion injury, or a gradual onset of low-grade pain through overuse.

On examination, the symptoms are reproduced by resisted eversion. In acute tenosynovitis, passive inversion may also be painful as the tendons are pulled through their inflamed sheath.

Treatment by injection

Corticosteroid injection into the shared synovial sheath or into the teno-osseous junction of peroneus brevis at the base of the fifth metatarsal may be curative. Alternative treatment may be by physiotherapeutic modalities including mobilization by transverse friction massage and electrotherapy (Cyriax & Cyriax 1983, Cyriax 1984, Kesson & Atkins 1998).

Needle size	25 G × $^5/_8$ in (0.5 × 16 mm) orange needle (teno-osseous junction) or 23 G × 1 in (0.6 × 25 mm) blue needle (tendons in sheath).

Dose	10 mg triamcinolone acetonide, 0.75 ml local anaesthetic, e.g. 0.25 ml Kenalog®, 0.75 ml 1% lidocaine.

Patient position

Position the patient supine in half lying, with the foot supported.

Palpation

Locate the lesion by palpation. If tenosynovitis is the lesion, the tendons run in a shared sheath behind and below the lateral malleolus. The peroneal tubercle (one finger's breadth below and anterior to the lateral malleolus) marks the distal end of the sheath and the point at which the tendons separate. Find the peroneal tubercle and mark a point between the two tendons.

If the lesion is at the insertion (teno-osseous junction) of peroneus brevis, locate the base of the fifth metatarsal and mark the tender point.

Technique

For tenosynovitis, insert the needle at the distal end of the shared sheath (see above); angle it posteriorly and between the peroneal tendons (Figs 10.21 and 10.22). Deliver the injection as a bolus into the shared sheath.

CLINICAL TIP: If tenosynovitis is due to inversion sprain, treatment using physiotherapeutic modalities such as friction massage and mobilization usually achieves excellent results (Cyriax & Cyriax 1983, Cyriax 1984, Kesson & Atkins, 1998).

For tendinitis at the teno-osseous junction of peroneus brevis, deliver the injection by a peppering technique at the area marked as tender at the base of the fifth metatarsal (Figs 10.23 and 10.24).

Patient advice

Advise the patient to maintain a period of relative rest for up to 2 weeks following the injection.

▶ FIGURE 10.21

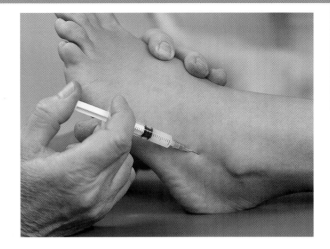

▶ FIGURE 10.22

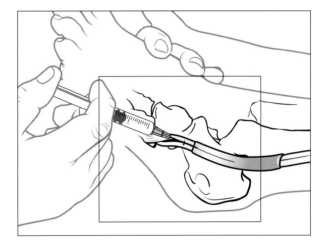

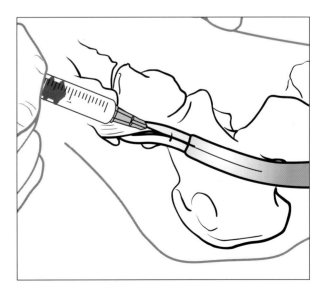

▶ **FIGURE 10.23**

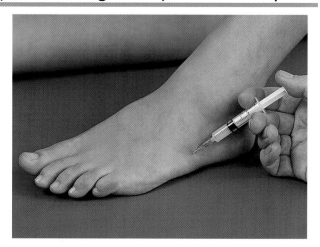

▶ **FIGURE 10.24**

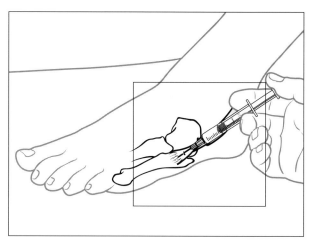

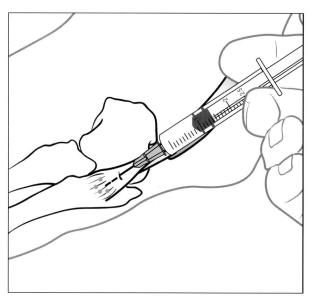

ACHILLES TENDON

Indication

Achilles tendinitis, which may respond well to corticosteroid injection, provided it involves early reversible inflammation of the paratenon. If the lesion becomes chronic, irreversible degenerative changes supersede the inflammatory changes and tendinosis is the main problem, i.e. focal degeneration (Williams 1986b, Mahler & Fritschy 1992). The lesion may be further complicated by partial or complete rupture.

Causes of Achilles tendinitis range from altered lower limb biomechanics, overpronation, ill-fitting footwear, pressure from heel counters and inappropriate or excessive training regimes, to an association with rheumatoid arthritis and the spondyloarthropathies (Smart et al 1980).

Patient presentation

The patient complains of a gradual onset of pain localized to the posterior aspect of the heel. Characteristically, pain and stiffness is present on first putting the foot to the floor after a night's rest, but this subsides after a few steps. The posterior location of the pain differentiates Achilles tendinitis from plantar fasciitis. The symptoms are aggravated by activity.

On examination, the affected area of the tendon may be observed as thickened. Resisted plantarflexion, particularly against the patient's bodyweight and gravity, reproduces the symptoms.

Treatment by injection

Conflicting evidence exists over the use of corticosteroid injections and their relationship to tendon rupture (Kennedy & Baxter Willis 1976, Smart et al 1980, Kleinman & Gross 1983, Mahler & Fritschy 1992, Read & Motto 1992, Maffulli 1999). Early Achilles tendinitis, involving inflammation of the paratenon, should respond well to corticosteroid injection alongside, **NOT INTO** the body of the tendon, but vigorous activity should be avoided for at least two weeks following the injection (Maffulli, 1999). Chronic lesions of tendinosis, where degeneration is the main feature, may not respond so readily and are prone to rupture whether or not they are injected. It remains questionable that rupture is due to a steroid effect or further manifestation of degenerate disease (Phelps et al 1974). Ultrasound scanning can help to establish degenerative changes and partial tears within the tendon, especially if a tender focal nodule is palpable.

Since one of the effects of corticosteroid injection is to weaken collagen fibres initially, the enforcement of relative rest after injection is of paramount importance to prevent this complication.

| **Needle size** | 21 G × 1½ in (0.8 × 40 mm) green needle. |

Dose	20 mg triamcinolone acetonide, 1.5 ml local anaesthetic, e.g. 0.5 ml Kenalog®, 1.5 ml 1% lidocaine.

Patient position

Position the patient in prone lying, with the lower leg supported and the ankle maintained in dorsiflexion.

Palpation

Two insertions need to be made, therefore palpate the distal tendon for the tenderness and mark a point on both sides of the tendon.

Technique

CLINICAL TIP: Bend the needle slightly at the hub, using the needle sheath to achieve this, to facilitate the injection parallel to the tendon.

Insert the needle to one side of, and parallel to, the Achilles tendon, advancing it to its full length (Figs 10.25, 10.26, 10.27 and 10.28). Deliver the injection as a bolus, depositing half the solution as the needle is withdrawn. Replace the needle and inject the remaining solution on the other side.

CLINICAL TIP: As a weight-bearing tendon and with the likelihood of degenerative changes within the tendon predisposing it to rupture, this injection technique aims to 'bathe' the tendon in corticosteroid solution and is **NOT** an injection into the body of the tendon itself.

Patient advice

Advise the patient to maintain a period of relative rest for up to 2 weeks after the injection. This is most important for the Achilles tendon since it is a weight-bearing tendon, and any possible weakening of the collagen fibre content of the tendon could predispose it to rupture. The causative factors need to be addressed and a heel-raise or orthotics may be appropriate.

▶ **FIGURE 10.25**

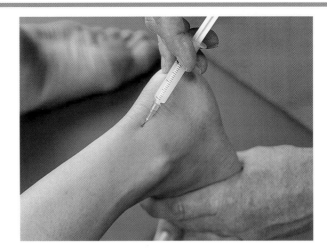

▶ **FIGURE 10.26**

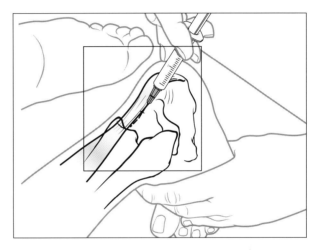

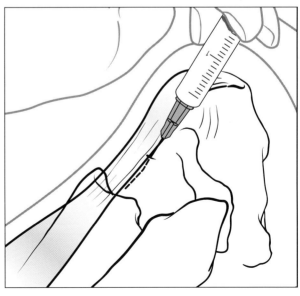

▶ **FIGURE 10.27**

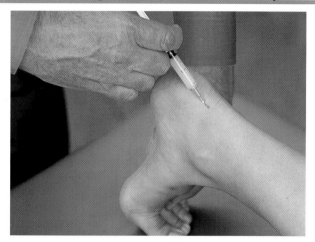

▶ **FIGURE 10.28**

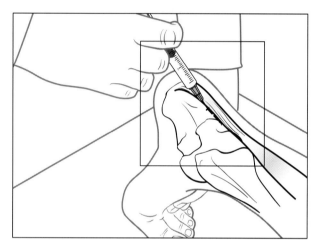

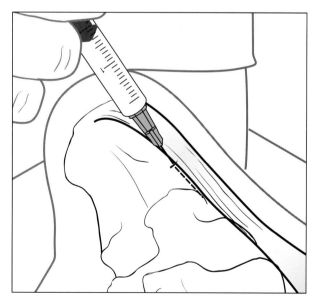

CONCLUSION

Section 2 has adopted a regional approach in presenting injection techniques for the treatment of peripheral musculoskeletal lesions. The upper limb lesions have been covered first, working through the shoulder, elbow and wrist and hand regions. Lower limb lesions follow, relating to the hip, knee and ankle and foot regions.

A consistent format has been used for each injection, providing details of indications, presentation, needle size, dosage, patient position, accurate palpation of the site, specific technique for the injection and the appropriate aftercare advice for the patient.

Guidelines for injection doses have been given throughout and it has been highlighted that the guidance for the dosage of steroid refers to the use of triamcinolone acetonide as an example, with the advice to consult the manufacturer's data sheet if another steroid is to be used.

The necessity for the use of a 'no touch' technique when injecting has been emphasized and *Clinical tips* have been offered both to ensure safety and to enhance effectiveness.

References

Anderson B, Kaye S 1991 Treatment for flexor tenosynovitis of the hand with corticosteroids. Archives of International Medicine 151(1): 153–156

Anton H A 1993 Frozen shoulder. Canadian Family Physician 39: 1773–1777

Apter A J, LaVallee H A 1994. How is anaphylaxis recognized? Archives of Family Medicine 3: 717–722

Armstrong P, Saxton H 1972 Ilio-psoas bursa. British Journal of Rheumatology 45: 493–495

Assendelft W J J, Hay E M, Adshead R, Bouter L M 1996 Corticosteroid injections for lateral epicondylitis: a systematic overview. British Journal of General Practice 46: 209–216

Association of the British Pharmaceutical Industry (ABPI) 2000 Compendium of Data Sheets and Summaries of Product Characteristics 1999–2000. Datapharm Publications Ltd, London

Baxter D E 1994 The heel in sport. Clinics in Sports Medicine 113: 683–693

Benet L 1996. General Principles. In: Hardman J G et al (eds) Goodman and Gilman's The Pharmacological Basis of Therapeutics, 9th edn. McGraw-Hill, New York

Bergman B 1990 Professional role and autonomy in physiotherapy. Scandinavian Journal of Rehabilitation and Medicine 22: 79–84

British National Formulary (BNF) 2000 British National Formulary, 39th edn. British Medical Association and Royal Pharmaceutical Society of Great Britain, London

Brown A F T 1995 Anaphylactic shock: mechanisms and treatment. Journal of Accident and Emergency Medicine 12: 89–100

Cailliet R 1990 Soft Tissue Pain and Disability, 2nd edn. F A Davis

Cameron G 1995a Steroid arthropathy – myth or reality? Journal of Orthopaedic Medicine 17: 51–55

Cameron G 1995b The shoulder is a weight-bearing joint: implications for clinical practice. Journal of Orthopaedic Medicine 17: 46–50

Carrico T J, Mehrhof A I, Cohen I K 1984 Biology of wound healing. Surgical Clinics of North America 64: 721–731.

Cawley P J, Morris I M 1992 A study to compare the efficacy of two methods of skin preparation prior to joint injection. British Journal of Rheumatology 31: 847–848.

Chakravarty K, Pharoah P D 1994 A randomised controlled study of post-injection rest following intra-articular steroid therapy for knee synovitis. British Journal of Rheumatology 33 (5): 464–468

Chartered Society of Physiotherapy (CSP) 1999 Clinical Guideline for the Use of Injection Therapy by Physiotherapists. CSP, London

Cohen I K, Diegelmann R F, Johnson M L 1977 Effect of corticosteroids on collagen synthesis. Surgery 82: 15–20.

Committee on Safety of Medicines (CSM) 1995 Tendon damage associated with quinolone antibiotics. HMSO, London

Coombs G M, Bax D E 1996 The use and abuse of steroids in rheumatology. Reports on Rheumatic Diseases Practical Problems Series 3. Arthritis and Rheumatism Council 8(3)

Coonrad R W, Hooper W R 1973 Tennis elbow: its course, natural history, conservative and surgical management. Journal of Bone and Joint Surgery 55-A: 1177–1182

Cooper C, Kirwan J R 1990 The risks of local and systemic corticosteroid administration. Baillière's Clinical Rheumatology 4(2): 305–332

Creamer P 1999 Intra-articular corticosteroid treatment in osteoarthritis. Current Opinion in Rheumatology 11(5): 417–421

Crown J 1999 The Crown Review of Prescribing, Supply and Administration of Medicines. Department of Health, London

Curwin S, Stanish W D 1984 Jumper's knee. In: Tendinitis – Its Aetiology and Treatment. Collamore Press, Oxford

Cyriax J 1982 Textbook of Orthopaedic Medicine, Vol 1, 8th edn. Baillière Tindall, London

Cyriax J 1984 Textbook of Orthopaedic Medicine, vol 2, 11th edn. Baillière Tindall, London

Cyriax J, Cyriax P 1983 Illustrated Manual of Orthopaedic Medicine. Butterworths, London

Dacre J E, Beeney N, Scott D L 1989 Injections and physiotherapy for the painful stiff shoulder. Annals of the Rheumatic Diseases 48: 322–325

Dasgupta B, Bowles J 1995 Scintigraphic localisation of steroid injection site in plantar fasciitis. Lancet 346: 1400–1401

De Jong B A, Dahmen R, Hogeweg J A, Marti R K 1998 Intra-articular triamcinolone acetonide injection in patients with capsulitis of the shoulder: a comparative study of two dose regimes. Clinical Rehabilitation 12 (3): 211–215

Dieppe P 1995 Management of hip osteoarthritis. British Medical Journal 311: 853–857

Dieppe P A, Sathapatayovongs H E, Jones P A, Bacon P A, Ring E F J 1980 Intra-articular steroids in osteoarthritis. Rheumatology and Rehabilitation 19: 212–217

Discussion Document 1988 The practice of physiotherapy. Physiotherapy 74: 356–358

Discussion Document 1990 The use of injections by physiotherapists. Physiotherapy 76: 218–219

Drugs and Therapeutics Bulletin 1995 Articular and peri-articular corticosteroid injections. Drugs and Therapeutics Bulletin 33(9): 67–70

Ehrlich H P, Hunt T K 1968 Effects of cortisone and vitamin A on wound healing. Annals of Surgery 167: 324–328

Ehrlich H P, Tarver H, Hunt T K 1972 Effects of vitamin A and glucocorticoids upon inflammation and collagen synthesis. Annals of Surgery 177: 222–227

Elliott B G 1992 Finkelstein's test: a descriptive error that can produce a false positive. Journal of Hand Surgery 17B: 481–482

Ernst E 1992 Conservative therapy for tennis elbow. British Journal of Clinical Practice 46: 55–57

Evans P 1990 Clinical biomechanics of the subtalar joint. Physiotherapy 76: 47–81

Flanagan F L, Sant S, Coughlan R J, O'Connell D 1995 Symptomatic enlarged iliopsoas bursae in the presence of a normal plain hip radiograph. British Society for Rheumatology 34: 365–369

Foley A E 1993 Tennis elbow. American Family Physician 48: 281–288

Frey C, Rosenberg Z, Shereff M J, Kim H 1992 The retrocalcaneal bursa: anatomy and bursography. Foot and Ankle 13: 203–207

Gabbott D A, Baskett P J F 1997 Management of the airway and ventilation during resuscitation. British Journal of Anaesthesia 79(2): 159–171

Gam A N, Schydlowsky P, Rossel I, Remvig L, Jensen E M 1998 Treatment of "frozen shoulder" with distension and glucocorticoid compared with glucocorticoid alone, a randomised controlled trial. Scandinavian Journal of Rheumatology 27(6): 425–430

Gellman H 1992 Tennis elbow (lateral epicondylitis). Orthopaedic Clinics of North America 23: 75–82

Gibbon W W, Cassar-Pullicino V N 1994 Heel pain. Annals of the Rheumatic Diseases 54: 344–348

Gilberthorpe J 1996 Problems in general practice – consent to treatment. Medical Defence Union, London

Grillet B, Dequeker J 1990 Intra-articular steroid injection – a risk–benefit assessment. Drug Safety 5(3): 205–211

Grubbs N 1993 Frozen shoulder syndrome – a review of the literature. Journal of Orthopaedics and Sports Physical Therapy 18: 479–487

Grundy H F 1990 Lecture Notes on Pharmacology, 2nd edn. Blackwell Scientific Publications, Oxford

Haker E, Lundeberg T 1993 Elbow-band, splintage and steroids in lateral epicondylalgia (tennis elbow). The Pain Clinic 6(2): 103–112

Handley J A 1997 Basic Life Support. British Journal of Anaesthesia 79(2): 151–158

Haslock I, MacFarlane D, Speed C 1995 Intra-articular and soft tissue injections: a survey of current practice. British Journal of Rheumatology 34: 449–452

Hattam P, Smeatham A 1999 Evaluation of an orthopaedic screening service in Primary Care. British Journal of Clinical Governance. 4: 45–49

Hay E M, Paterson S, Lewis M et al 1999 Pragmatic randomised controlled trial of local corticosteroid injection and naproxen for treatment of lateral epicondylitis of elbow in primary care. British Medical Journal 319: 964–968

Henry J 1991 The British Medical Association Guide to Medicines and Drugs, 2nd edn. Dorling Kindersley, London

Hockin J, Bannister G 1994 The extended role of a physiotherapist in an outpatient orthopaedic clinic. Physiotherapy 80: 281–284

Hollingworth G R, Ellis R, Hattersley T S 1983 Comparison of injection techniques for shoulder pain: results of a double blind, randomised study. British Medical Journal 287: 1339–1341

Hoppenfeld S 1976 Physical Examination of the Spine and Extremities. Appleton Century Crofts.

Hourigan P G, Weatherley C R 1994 The physiotherapist as an orthopaedic assistant in a spinal clinic. Physiotherapy 80: 484

Hughes R A 1996 Septic arthritis. Reports on Rheumatic Diseases (Series 3), practical problems. Arthritis and Rheumatism Council

Hunter J A, Blyth T H 1999 A risk–benefit assessment of intra-articular corticosteroids in rheumatic disorders (review). Drug Safety 21(5): 353–365

Hutson M A 1990 Sports Injuries – Recognition and Management. Oxford Medical Publications.

Jacob A K, Sallay P I 1997 Therapeutic efficacy of corticosteroid injections in the acromioclavicular joint. Biomedical Sciences Instrumentation 34: 380–385

Jacobs L G H, Barton M A J, Wallace W A et al 1991 Intra-articular distension and steroids in the management of capsulitis of the shoulder. British Medical Journal 302: 1498–1501

Jones A, Regan M, Ledingham J, Pattrick M, Manhire A, Doherty M 1993 Importance of placement of intra-articular steroid injections. British Medical Journal 307: 1329–1330

Kalant H 1998 Introduction to General Pharmacology. In: Kalant H, Roschlau WHE (eds) Principles of Medical Pharmacology, 6th edn. Oxford University Press, New York

Karr S D 1994 Subcalcaneal heel pain. Orthopedic Clinics of North America 25: 161–175

Kennedy J C, Baxter Willis R 1976 The effects of local steroid injections on tendons: a biomechanical and microscopic correlative study. American Journal of Sports Medicine 4: 11–21

Kerlan R K, Glousman R E 1989 Injections and techniques in athletic medicine. Clinics in Sports Medicine 8 (3): 541–560

Kerry R, King D G, Gibson M F 2000 Iliopsoas bursitis: physical management with ultrasonography and corticosteroid infiltration in a 33 year-old man. Physiotherapy 86(6): 306–311

Kesson M, Atkins A 1998 Orthopaedic Medicine: a Practical Approach. Butterworth Heinemann, Oxford

Kibler W B, Goldberg C, Chandler T J 1991 Functional biomechanical deficits in running athletes with plantar fasciitis. American Journal of Sports Medicine 19: 66–71

Kleinman M, Gross A E 1983 Achilles tendon rupture following steroid injection. Journal of Bone and Joint Surgery 65-A: 1345–1347.

Klug J D 1995 MR diagnosis of tenosynovitis about the wrist. MRI Clinics of North America 3: 305–312

Korniewicz D M, Laughon B E, Butz A, Larson E 1989 Integrity of vinyl and latex procedure gloves. Nursing Research 38(3): 144–146

Kulick M I, Brazlow R, Smith S, Hentz V R 1984 Injectable ibuprofen: preliminary evaluation of its ability to decrease peritendinous adhesions. Annals of Plastic Surgery 13: 459–467

Kumar P, Clark M 1994 Clinical Medicine, 3rd edn. Baillière Tindall, London

Kumar N, Newman R J 1999 Complications of intra- and peri-articular steroid injections. British Journal of General Practice 49: 465–466

Lambert M A, Morton R J, Sloan J P 1992 Controlled study of the use of local steroid injection in the treatment of trigger finger and thumb. Journal of Hand Surgery 17B: 69–70

Laurence D R, Bennett P N, Brown M J 1997 Clinical Pharmacology, 8th edn. Churchill Livingstone, Edinburgh

Le Gros Clark, W E 1965 The Tissues of the Body, 5th edn. Oxford University Press, Oxford

Livengood L 1992 Occupational soft tissue disorders of the hand and forearm. Wisconsin Medical Journal: 583–584

Lloyd Davies A 1998 Adult trigger finger – a literature review of the aetiology and conservative treatment. Journal of Orthopaedic Medicine 20(3): 7–12

Mace S, Vadas P, Pruzanski W 1997 Anaphylactic shock induced by intra-articular injection of methylprednisolone acetate. Journal of Rheumatology 24(6): 1191–1194

Maffulli N 1999 Rupture of the Achilles tendon. The Journal of Bone and Joint Surgery 81-A(7): 1019–1036

Mahler F, Fritschy D 1992 Partial and complete ruptures of the Achilles tendon and local corticosteroid injections. British Journal of Sports Medicine 26: 7–13

Marks J G, Cano C, Leitzel K, Lipton A 1983 Inhibition of wound healing by topical steroids. Journal of Dermatological Surgery and Oncology 9: 819–821

Mazanec D J 1995 Pharmacology of corticosteroids in synovial joints. Physical Medicine and Rehabilitation Clinics of North America 6(4): 815–821

Meaney J F, Cassar-Pullicino V N, Ethrington R et al 1992 Ilio-psoas bursa enlargement. Clinical Radiology 45: 161–168

Millard R S, Dillingham M F 1995 Peripheral joint injections. Physical Medicine and Rehabilitation Clinics of North America 6(4): 841–849

Murphy D, Failla J M, Koniuch M P 1995 Steroid versus placebo injection for trigger finger. Journal of Hand Surgery 20A: 628–631

Nelson K H, Briner W, Cummins J 1995 Corticosteroid injection therapy for overuse injuries. American Family Physician 52(1): 1811–1816

Neustadt D H 1991 Local corticosteroid injection therapy in soft tissue rheumatic conditions of the wrist and hand. Arthritis and Rheumatism 34(7): 923–926

News Item 2000 Prescribing proposals for PTs. Frontline 6(5): 7

Norris C M 1993 Sports Injuries: Diagnosis and Management for Physiotherapists. Butterworth Heinemann, London

Noteboom T, Cruver R, Keller J et al 1994 Tennis elbow: a review. Journal of Orthopaedic and Sports Physical Therapy 19: 357–366

Otto N, Wehbé M A 1986 Steroid injections for tenosynovitis in the hand. Orthopaedic Review 15(5): 45–48

Pal B, Morris J 1999 Perceived risks of joint infection following intra-articular corticosteroid injections: a survey of rheumatologists. Clinical Rheumatology 18(3): 264–265

Parikh J R, Houpt J B, Jacobs S, Fernandes B J 1993 Charcot's arthropathy of the shoulder following intra-articular corticosteroid injections. Journal of Rheumatology 20: 885–887

Palve H, Kirvela O H, Olin H, Syvalahti E, Kanto J 1995 Maximum recommended doses of lignocaine are not toxic. British Journal of Anaesthesia 74(6): 704–705

Pfenninger J L 1991 Injections of joints and soft tissues. Part 1. General guidelines. American Family Physician 44: 1196–1202

Pfizer Pharmaceuticals 1996 Joint Injection Techniques: a User's Guide. Pfizer Pharmaceuticals, Sandwich

Phelps S, Sonstegard D A, Matthews L S 1974 Corticosteroid injection effects on the biomechanical properties of rabbit patellar tendons. Clinical Orthopaedics and Related Research 100: 345–348

Ponec M, de Haas C, Bachra B N, Polano M K 1997 Effects of glucocorticoids on primary human skin fibroblasts. Research 117–123

Price R, Sinclair H, Heinrich I, Gibson T 1991 Local injection treatment of tennis elbow-hydrocortisone, triamcinolone and lidocaine compared. British Journal of Rheumatology 30: 39–44

Rang H O, Dale M M, Ritter J M 1995 Pharmacology. 3rd edn. Churchill Livingstone, Edinburgh

Rasmussen K J E, Fano N 1985 Trochanteric bursitis: treatment by corticosteroid injection. Scandinavian Journal of Rheumatology 14: 417–420

Read M T F, Motto S G 1992 Tendo Achilles pain: steroids and outcome. British Journal of Sports Medicine 26: 15–21

Rettig A 1994 Wrist problems in the tennis player. Medicine and Science in Sports and Exercise 26: 1207–1212

Rifat S F, Moeller J L 2001 Site-specific techniques of joint injection. Useful additions to your treatment repertoire. Postgraduate Medicine 109(3): 123–136

Salisbury D M, Begg N T 1996 Immunisation against infectious disease. HMSO, London

Sambrook P N, Champion G D, Browne C D et al 1989 Corticosteroid injection for osteoarthritis of the knee: peripatellar compared with intra-articular route. Clinical and Experimental Rheumatology 7: 609–613

Sandberg N 1964 Time relationship between administration of cortisone and wound healing in rats. Acta Chirurgiae Scandinavica 127: 446–455

Saunders S, Cameron G 1997 Injection techniques in orthopaedic and sports medicine. Saunders and Co, London

Schapira D, Nahir M, Scharf Y 1986 Trochanteric bursitis: a common clinical problem. Arch Phys Med Rehabil 67: 815–817

Schimmer B P, Parker K L 1996 Adrenocorticotrophic hormone; Adrenocortical steroids and their synthetic analogues; inhibitors of the synthesis and actions of adrenocortical hormones. In: Hardman J G et al (eds) Goodman and Gilman's The Pharmacological Basis of Therapeutics, 9th edn. McGraw-Hill, New York

Schimmer B P, George S R 1998 Adrenocortical Steroid Hormones. In: Kalant H, Roschlau W H E (eds) Principles of Medical Pharmacology, 6th edn. Oxford University Press, New York

Scott D B 1989 Editorial 'Maximum recommended doses' of local anaesthetic drugs. British Journal of Anaesthesia 63(4): 373

Sellman J R 1994 Plantar fascia rupture associated with corticosteroid injection. Foot and Ankle International 15: 376–381

Shbeeb M I, O'Duffy J D, Michet Jr C J, O'Fallon W M, Matteson E L 1996 Evaluation of glucocorticosteroid injection for the treatment of trochanteric bursitis. The Journal of Rheumatology 23(12): 2104–2106

Shea K G, Shumsky I B, Shea O F 1991 Shifting wrist pain – de Quervain's disease and off-road biking. Physician and Sports Medicine 19: 59–63

Silver T 1999 Joint and Soft Tissue Injection. Radcliffe Medical Press, Abingdon

Singh D, Angel J, Bentley G, Trevino S G 1997 Plantar fasciitis. British Medical Journal 315: 172–175

Smart G W, Taunton J E, Clement D B 1980 Achilles tendon disorders in runners – a review. Medicine and Science in Sports and Exercise 12: 231–243

Smith D L, Wernick R 1994 Common nonarticular syndromes in the elbow, wrist and hand. Postgraduate Medicine 95: 1173–1188

Sölveborn, S-A, Buch F, Mallmin H, Adalberth G 1995 Corticosteroid injection with anaesthetic additives for radial epicondylalgia (tennis elbow). Clinical Orthopaedics and Related Research 316: 99–105

Speed CA 2001 Corticosteroid injection in tendon lesions. British Medical Journal 323: 382–386

Stahl S, Kaufman T 1997 Ulnar nerve injury at the elbow after steroid injection for medial epicondylitis. Journal of Hand Surgery 22B(1): 69–70

Stam H W 1994 Frozen shoulder – a review of current concepts. Physiotherapy 80: 588–598

Stearns M L 1940a Studies on the development of connective tissue in transparent chambers in the rabbit's ear, I. American Journal of Anatomy 66: 133–176

Stearns M L 1940b Studies on the development of connective tissue in transparent chambers in the rabbit's ear, II. American Journal of Anatomy 67: 55–97

Stefanich R J 1986 Intra-articular corticosteroids in the treatment of osteoarthritis. Orthopaedic Review 15(2): 27–33

Stephens M M 1994 Haglund's deformity and retrocalcaneal bursitis. Orthopaedic Clinics of North America 25: 41–46

Sutton G 1984 Hamstrung by hamstring strains: a review of the literature. Journal of Orthopaedics and Sports Physical Therapy 5: 184–195

Swain R A, Kaplan B. 1995 Practices and pitfalls of corticosteroid injection. The Physician and Sports Medicine 23(3): 27–40

Tan M Y, Low C K, Tan S K 1994 De Quervain's tenosynovitis and ganglion over the first dorsal extensor retinacular compartment. Annals Academy of Medicine 23: 885–886

Toohey A K, LaSalle T L, Martinez S, Polisson R P 1990 Iliopsoas bursitis: clinical features, radiographic findings, and disease associations. Seminars in Arthritis and Rheumatism 20: 41–47

Underwood P L, McLeod R A, Ginsburg W W 1988 The varied clinical manifestations of iliopsoas bursitis. Journal of Rheumatology 18: 1810–1812

Van der Heijden G J M G, van der Windt D A W M, Kleijnen J et al 1996 Steroid injections for shoulder disorders: a systematic review of randomized clinical trials. British Journal of General Practice 46: 309–316

Van der Windt D A, Koes B W, Deville W et al 1998 Effectiveness of corticosteroid injections versus physiotherapy for the treatment of painful stiff shoulder in primary care: randomised trial. British Medical Journal 317 (7168): 1292–1296

Vargas Busquets M A V 1994 Historical commentary: the wrist flexion test (Phalen's sign). Journal of Hand Surgery 19: 521

Verhaar J A N, Walenkamp G H I M, van Mameren H et al 1996 Local corticosteroid injection versus Cyriax-type physiotherapy for tennis elbow. Journal of Bone and Joint Surgery 78-B: 128–132

Weitoft T, Uddenfeldt P 2000 Importance of synovial fluid aspiration when injecting intra-articular corticosteroids. Annals of the Rheumatic Diseases 59 (3): 233–235

Williams J 1986a Physiotherapy is handling. Physiotherapy 75: 66–70

Williams J G P 1986b Achilles tendon lesions in sport. Sports Medicine 3: 114–115

Williams P L, Warwick R, Dyson M, Bannister L H 1989 Gray's Anatomy, 37th edn. Churchill Livingstone

Wood-Smith F G, Stewart H C, Vickers M D 1968 Drugs in Anaesthetic Practice. 3rd edn. Butterworths, London

Wyatt R 1996 Anaphylaxis: How to recognize, treat, and prevent potentially fatal attacks. Postgraduate Medicine 100(2): 87–99

Appendix

The **capsular pattern** is a limitation of movement in a specific pattern that is peculiar to each joint, and is a useful finding for clinical diagnosis since it indicates the presence of an arthritis. The pattern varies from joint to joint and is characterized by limitation of movement in a fixed proportion. It is the same whatever the cause of the arthritis (Cyriax 1982, Cyriax & Cyriax 1983) and the history and investigations will suggest and lead to confirmation of the specific form. The movements that become limited in the capsular pattern take on a defined 'hard' end-feel.

Capsular patterns

Joint	Capsular pattern
Shoulder joint	Most limitation of lateral rotation followed by abduction Least limitation of medial rotation
Elbow joint	More limitation of flexion than extension
Radio-ulnar joint	Pain at end of range of both rotatons
Wrist joint	Equal limitation of flexion and extension Eventual fixation in the mid-position
Trapezio-first metacarpal joint	Most limitation of extension
Metacarpophalangeal joints	Limitation of radial deviation and extension
Interphalangeal joints	Equal limitation of flexion and extension
Hip joint	Most limitation of medial rotation followed by limitation of flexion and abduction Eventual limitation of extension
Knee joint	More limitation of flexion than extension
Ankle joint	More limitation of plantarflexion than dorsiflexion
Subtalar joint	Increasing limitation of supination Eventual fixation in pronation
Midtarsal joint	Limitation of adduction and supination Forefoot fixes in abduction and pronation
First metatarsophalangeal joint	Gross limitation of extension Some limitation of flexion
Other metatarsophalangeal joints	May vary: usually more limitation of flexion and extension
Interphalangeal joints	Fix in flexion

Index

Page numbers in **bold** refer to major musculoskeletal lesions/regions which include patient presentation, needle size, dose, patient position, palpation and injection technique.